THE STORY OF A
PRUDENT
NURSE

THE STORY OF A
PRUDENT NURSE

A Heartwarming Memoir with Krysha
and May Cabuenas-Clemente

JOEL J. CLEMENTE
With Krysha Clemente and May Cabuenas-Clemente

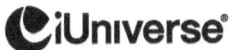

THE STORY OF A PRUDENT NURSE
A Heartwarming Memoir with Krysha
and May Cabuenas-Clemente

iUniverse books may be ordered through booksellers or by contacting:

iUniverse
1663 Liberty Drive
Bloomington, IN 47403
www.iuniverse.com
1-800-Authors (1-800-288-4677)

ISBN: 978-1-5320-2676-8 (sc)
ISBN: 978-1-5320-2677-5 (e)

Library of Congress Control Number: 2017910024

Print information available on the last page.

iUniverse rev. date: 07/03/2017

To the Holy Trinity, Father, Son, and Holy Spirit;
to the Holy Family, St. Joseph, the Blessed Virgin Mary,
and Jesus; and to the people who I am called to serve

Recipient

A portion of the proceeds from *The Story of a Prudent Nurse* will go to the Ateneo de Zamboanga University College of Nursing Scholarship Fund, Jesuit Volunteers Philippines Foundation Inc., and St. Gabriel the Archangel Catholic Community.

CONTENTS

FOREWORD
BY FATHER CYRAIN CABUENAS

At the outset, one may think that this book is an against-all-odds story of a nurse who searched for a greener pasture and through sheer guts and grit, clawed his way to the top. Actually, it is but so much more. That's why somehow, this book is a vade mecum for those immigrants and their families who are scattered by economic necessity and want to fulfill their American dream.

This is all the more compelling because it shows the powerful sentiments and deep attachments of the author to his family and his nostalgic reflections on how he carried his burden with patience and dignity. More importantly, it talks about his moving personal journey of faith and how his trust in the Divine Providence did not break his heart or his resolve.

I have known the author for quite sometime now. Actually, he is my favorite brother-in-law, since I have only one sister. Looking back, I have always known him to be a man on a mission, a man for others. Perhaps, it was his Jesuit education. That's why it doesn't come as a surprise that he would go out of his way to help those in need as the one plane incident in his book fittingly describes his altruism.

Despite the privileges and the perks that come with citizenship and stable job, I am privy to the simplicity of the author's household. Excess is alien. His monicker – prudent nurse – fits. But I also know how extravagant and lavish his heart and his dreams are. Irresistibly, his passion for writing paid off and he found his way to express himself without pretense tjhrough this remarkable book that we can all resonate with.

NOTES FROM THE FAMILY OF JOEL J. CLEMENTE

"Kuya Jong" as we fondly call him, is an opinionated writer who speaks his mind in a variety field of interests. His versatile talent in writing touches poetry, personal views on social and work issues, newsletters and in almost any genre in which he pours his heart out. Reading his works, you will laugh and cry; object and emphathize with him; be entertained and moved. All of these compel you to read his book and make it a part of your coffee table collection.

-Father Clyde Cabuenas
Former Seminary Formator and Professor in Philosophy
Philippine Daily Inquirer Visayas Bureau

Joel is the type of person who can stand up tall and who keeps moving forward despite the trials that came his way. He is resilient and driven to reach his dreams. I was a witness to this, and it is indeed inspiring. Continue with what you have started, Joel. Be of service to others while trusting in God. Keep it up, Jong!

—Lilian Lourdes Clemente-Ballelos

Being the second youngest of eleven children, Joel had to face many challenges and deal with the many different and strong personalities of his siblings. He also had to live up to the expectations of others that he complete at least four years of college. These life experiences must have helped him maintain balance in his personal life.

The most important attribute in Joel's success in life is his *perseverance.* While in the Philippines, he was determined to come to the United States—eager to advance his career in nursing and allow him and his family the opportunity to pursue the American dream.

He knew that passing the Commission of Graduates of Foreign Nursing Schools (CGFNS) was a requirement and stepping-stone for a nursing career in the United States. For ten years, at the cost of several thousand dollars, he struggled to pass it, leaving him and his family extremely disappointed and him in debt. But he continued to pursue his dream, finally passing it and moving to the United States. The hardships he experienced must have been an inspiration, teaching him and his family to *never* give up.

—Mary Jacqueline Clemente-Yeosock

ACKNOWLEDGMENTS

The publication of this book was made possible through the following people and groups, who encouraged me, inspired me, and helped me put together the pieces of my life's journey for God and country:

Father Clyde Cabuenas
Father Cyrain Cabuenas
Mr. and Mrs. Lucio Cabuenas
Ms. Krysha May Clemente
Mrs. May Cabuenas-Clemente
Mr. Enrique Clemente
Mrs. Grace Jones-Clemente
Rainier and Tessie Clemente and family
Helen Grace and Nonoy Elopre and family
Enrique Jr. and Edna Clemente and family
Mary Jacqueline and Michael Yeosock and family
Rommel and Leonora Clemente and family
Alexander and Archel Clemente and family
Rameses and Neneng Clemente and family
Jennifer and James See and family
Lilian Lourdes and Manuelito Ballelos and family
Amapola and Elmer Tamayo and family
Father Charles Githinji

Mr. Dave Manders
Father Jim Sichko
Father Romeo Solidon
Father Don Zeiler

Angkong Kiddos
Ateneo de Zamboanga University (ADZU) BSN Plexus
    1990 batch mates and mentors
ADZU College Beacon Yearbook Editorial Staff (ES)
ADZU College of Nursing *Pacemaker Nursing Magazine* (ES)
Armed Forces of the Philippines Medical Center (AFPMC)
AFPMC Newsletter (ES)
Genesis HealthCare Heritage Hall North, South and
    West Nursing Staff (NS)
Horizon Recruitment Pacific Corporation
Kindred Hospital Dallas Central (NS)
Friends of Mercy
Jesuit Volunteers Philippines (JVP) Foundation Inc.
JVP 11 (1990/1991) batch mates and formation staff
National Shrine of the Divine Mercy
Pinoy Elite at Westridge
St. Gabriel the Archangel Catholic community
St. Gabriel's Christ Renews His Parish fellow alumni
St. Gabriel's Hospitality Ministry Team
St. Gabriel's Knights of Columbus council
St. Gabriel's Men's Club
Sulat Town Folks
WorldWide HealthStaff Associates Ltd.

POINT OF VIEW BY KRYSHA MAY CLEMENTE

As Joel Clemente's daughter, it's been a great honor and a privilege to have the opportunity to be part of the making of this book written by my dad, Jong, in coordination with my mom, May, and two uncles, who were witnesses to his creativity in writing. Not only was it a gargantuan work to be part of, but said book also speaks what's in the heart and mind of my dad's journey.

Dad's love for freelance writing started thirty-one years ago when he was a senior student in high school back in our home country, the Philippines. From that day on, he wrote anything under the sun, from essays, short stories, poems, and feature news articles to testimonial stories—all of which he offered to God. He inherited this talent from his father, my *lolo*, a.k.a. Grandfather Enrique, who was a prolific writer during his time.

With almost a hundred manuscripts under his belt, his "small success" as a writer—as he framed it—came in the form of recognition by the public. This recognition, in both online and print publications, was evidenced by good comments and reviews. For some of this writing, he was even financially compensated for a job well done.

Besides being a down-to-earth, simple writer, my dad is a good, kind, loving, and responsible husband to my mom and father to me. We are truly blessed and proud to have him in our family. The energy and stamina he had to combine three roles at the same time—that of a nurse, a writer, and a volunteer—is beyond compare. And it's a true testament of his being a man for others.

I learned from him the value of "living simply so that others may simply live" and to continue to always be a "blessing to everyone." More so, he taught me to always look for the goodness and kindness of other people, regardless of color, race, and socioeconomic status.

Hence, while it is true that this book may or may not make you happy or sad, somehow you will join my dad's life journey as you read and ponder from page to page. You will discover that, in all the things that he does, he always puts the Divine Providence, as well as our family, at the top of his priorities. Both have positively influenced him. We hope reading about this journey, as you figure out what's the inside story of this book, may positively influence you.

INTRODUCTION BY
MAY CABUENAS-CLEMENTE

The pen is mightier than the sword.

It is with great joy that I present to you *The Story of a Prudent Nurse*. It captures the journey of my friend, hubby, and partner, Jong—as a prudent nurse, a freelance writer, and a community service volunteer—through several articles that he wrote through the years. Most of these articles were published in leading local and national nursing journals, magazines, and newsletters, both in the Philippines and in this great nation.

Part 1 shares his opinions and views on matters affecting the nursing profession that readers will find worth discussing.

Part 2 contains essays and testimonials from his college days, including his winning essay, graduation wishes, summer vacation notes, and a piece on working in a skilled nursing facility. It addresses also the power of prayers in our lives and shows how he went above and beyond the call of duty. This part also includes our family's testimonial story. It shows how we moved to this country after years of hardships and struggles. And it contains his colorful and meaningful narration of our daughter's life story.

Part 3 highlights him being featured in a critical care nursing journal, where he shared his tales as a staff nurse. This section has a great impact on his success.

Part 4 tackles his dual role as a class representative and historian, respectively. In this capacity, he wrote the colorful history of the college's BSN Plexus 1990 group in celebration of their twenty-fifth anniversary alumni homecoming reunion.

Part 5 contains three of his unforgettable literary poems. One poem depicts the message of the first Christmas. The second lists the qualities of a prudent nurse. And the last one contains reflections of a writer on things that have a bearing to significant human experiences.

Part 6 includes recognitions he received from numerous institutions, including his alma mater, Genesis HealthCare, and American Airlines, as a resident and an administrator. All of these are manifestations of his writing excellence and portray him as he has always been—a service-oriented person caring for other people.

We hope that this book will be the kind of book that you enjoy reading. After all, the purpose of *The Story of a Prudent Nurse* is to share with you Jong's experiences and lessons in life that makes him a radical and unique individual in loving service to God and others.

PART I

COMMENTARIES

CHAPTER 1

QUESTIONS OF THE MONTH

How could television improve its portrayal of nurses?[1]

Television's portrayal of nurses can improve by showing how nurses work for the good of everyone. In depicting this, television can help people understand that, despite the high cost of health care, providers like nurses are ready to lend a helping hand to assists patients in achieving an optimum level of functioning.

What is the most challenging aspect of your job?[2]

The ability to handle difficult patients, no matter what the situation is. This has given me the courage, strength, and stamina to cope with stress and tension—especially when schedules are too hectic and I need to make a firm decision in emergency cases. Moreover, it helps me to be

---

[1]   Original published in *RN Journal*, February 2007.
[2]   Original published in *RN Journal*, August 2008.

more caring and compassionate to patients, like I would be to a brother or friend. This helps them recover from their illnesses or helps them die with dignity and peace as the need arises.

CHAPTER 2

CHARTING CHALLENGES[3]

The June 13 cover story "Charting Challenges" is, indeed, an educational and interesting topic on computer literacy, especially for inexperienced nurses. Becoming computer savvy takes time and practice. And it really helps us to have more time with our patients. Less paperwork translates to the ability to give our best care to the people we serve.

I remember when I started working as a nurse in 1991. Charting was all paper-based and truly time-consuming. However, eighteen years later, when electronic record keeping was implemented in our facility, things changed. I saw the great differences between both forms of documentation.

---

[3] Original published in *Nurse.Com The Magazine, South*, August 8, 2011.

CHAPTER 3

HOW TO REDUCE THE ESCALATING SUICIDE RATE[4]

Since the time of Judas Iscariot and Socrates, suicide has been and still is one of the most tragic and disturbing incidents that could happen to a family or community. While its cause is complex and broad, the solution or prevention obviously requires a concerted effort from family members, institutions, policy makers, health workers, and other government agencies.

According to the World Health Organization, suicide rates all over the world have increased by 5 percent to 62 percent in the last two decades. One person commits suicide every 40 seconds. In the United States alone, there are eighty-three suicides per day or one in every seventeen minutes as reported by the American Association for Suicidology, and it's the eighth leading cause of death among Americans. The highest rates of cases are among

---

[4] Original report published in *Springfield Technical Community College Journal*, April 2008.

the elderly (sixty-five years old and over, especially those who are divorced or widowed) and the youth (fifteen to twenty-four years old).

The National Institute of Mental Health and the US Department of Health and Human Services identified the risk factors as depression and other mental disorders; substance abuse; family violence, including physical and sexual abuse, firearms; and economic or financial problems.

Surprisingly, the first world and developed countries are the leading contenders for highest rates of suicide and suicidal tendencies—Russia, Belgium, Austria, France, Switzerland, Denmark, Sweden, Australia, Canada, the United States, South Korea, and Japan. Except for in Russia, the happiness index in the aforementioned countries is quite high.

But then again, happiness attributed to wealth, success, or fame does not guarantee any antidote to taking one's life. One has only to recall the tragic cases of famous people, like Vincent van Gogh, Adolf Hitler, Jack London, Virginia Woolf, Marilyn Monroe, Kurt Cobain, and Chris Benoit.

Before we prescribe the preventive measures that reduce suicide rates, it might help if we tried to decipher first why we need to stop this act. We need to understand its sociological, cultural, and religious dimensions.

Psychologists assert that there is a suicidal tendency in almost every person, the longing for rest without conflicts. But some people are just plain nuts or mental cases. Two examples are Seung-Hui Cho, the gunman in the Virginia Tech massacre who shot himself after shooting to death thirty-two students, and Matthew J. Murray of the Colorado YWAM and New Life shootings.

Suicide should not be tolerated; it is a crime against a person's obligation toward his dependents and community. There is no self-made person. A person's growth, upbringing, and success can be traced to the efforts of other people. Suicide is a selfish and cowardly act. (Euthanasia for practical reasons and suicide of spies or soldiers to conceal secrets are different stories.)

Moreover, as a Christian, I believe the owner and master of one's life is God alone. Suicide is a total violation of the precepts of loving oneself and striving for perfection. In the early church years, a Christian burial was even denied to a suicide case.

For the Muslim extremists who continually detonate bombs attached to their bodies in Iraq and the terrorists who willfully crashed planes into the Twin Towers, suicide is ironically equivalent to martyrdom, sainthood, and heroism. Family members laud the action; no tears are shed; and, at times, there are even financial compensations.

For the majority who respect and enjoy life, suicide should be diminished and attempts should be nipped in the bud. Obviously, this is a responsibility not only of the government but also of almost every institution. Proper education and guidance is a must. The proficiency of health and welfare services should be increased. Crisis counseling organizations should be established. Domestic violence and substance abuse should be reduced, along with access to convenient means of suicide (handguns and toxic substances foremost).

The recession and financial crisis that we face these days may add to suicide rates, especially among those who cannot accept the prospect of leading a life without luxury and comfort. But I believe that depression, hopelessness, and failed relationships are greater contributors to this malady than is material loses. Thus, strengthening of family values should be the most important aspect. Statistics show that suicide rates are almost absent among happily married couples. Marital counseling and psychotherapy should be encouraged also. But it should be noted that even the father of psychotherapy, Sigmund Freud, committed suicide.

Proper FDA-approved medication for schizophrenic people, such as serotonin and clozapine, should also be applied. But such medications should be taken and given in moderation, unless one would like to end up like Heath Ledger.

References

World Health Organization data through the research of Chris Pearson

National Institute of Mental Health and US Department of Health and Human Services American Association for Suicidology

CHAPTER 4

RESOLVED THAT FILIPINO NURSES BE HIRED IN THE UNITED STATES OF AMERICA[5]

With the alarming shortages of nurses in the United States, the hiring of foreign nurses, including Filipino RNs, must transpire. This is no longer merely an option but, rather, an economic necessity due to rising population projections and a shrinking nursing workforce.

To start with, there is among the profession the perception that hiring Filipino nurses has several disadvantages. One contributing factor is the nationalistic attitude of Americans who are proud of their heritage and people and so believe the slots taken by Filipino nurses should have been given to natural born American nurses. Another factor is perception of a language barrier—the belief that Filipino nurses will have a hard time communicating with patients because English is not their forte. Thirdly, there is a notion that, because

---

[5]   Original report published in *Springfield Technical and Community College Journal*, November 2007.

of cultural differences, Filipino nurses will have a hard time adjusting to the progressive and liberal culture of the United States. Lastly is the belief that, due to climate and weather differences, Filipino nurses coming from a tropical country will have a hard time coping with the change of seasons, especially during wintertime.

However, recruiting Filipino nurses has some advantages. First, if America claims that the United States is the land of the free, then immigrants, like Filipino nurses who are qualified and deserving should be given a chance. Nationalism does not mean discrimination or narrow-mindedness, especially when diversifying the workforce can contribute to the economy and provide a substantial service. Moreover, the people of the United States should remember that theirs is a country of immigrants, a history that traces way back to the maiden voyage of the *Mayflower.* Therefore, America should also open her doors to other immigrants, including Filipino nurses.

Second, the perception that English is not a forte of Filipinos is entirely baseless and contradictory. English is the medium of instruction used at all the schools and universities in the Philippines. Moreover, English is also the primary language used in business transactions, all forms of media, and even in applying for jobs and at every formal gathering. While a number of Filipinos have thick accent and are guilty of grammar lapses, there is no place in the entirety of the 7,100 islands of the Philippines where English may sound Greek. Statistics show that Filipinos easily learn the different major languages all over the world because, in the Philippines alone, some 111 different dialects are spoken. To get by, one has only to talk in

English. In addition, statistics show that the Philippines is the third largest English-speaking nation in the world.

Third, yes, there may be cultural differences in terms of eating habits or lifestyle, but the culture of Filipinos, albeit traditional in some sense, could even be a plus factor. It is entirely ingrained in the value system of Filipinos to preserve, unite, and protect their families. The welfare of their loved ones is of paramount importance. It is almost an obligation to take care of the children and the elderly. The closely knit family ties are classic proof that no family member gives up on a family member. There is a maxim in the Philippines that states, "Blood is thicker than water." It means that, even if a family member or distant relative is not a good person, in times of trouble, he or she will find support from family members. Moreover, Filipinos never send their elderly to nursing homes. Parents or grandparents are cared for at home by their children or grandchildren. It is almost a crime if old folks are not given proper attention. One will get the ire of the neighbors and will be branded ungrateful if he or she takes the elderly for granted. Hence, Filipino nurses are a must in the United States; they know from experience how to take good care of the children and the elderly, and this knowledge will transfer to their treatment of the patients in their care.

Fourth, while it is true that Filipinos know only two seasons—dry and wet—that does not necessarily mean they cannot adjust to climate changes. Millions of Filipinos are working all over the world—some doing backbreaking jobs in the hottest of continents, like Africa or the Middle East. Others work on tankers and cruise ships that traverse the north and south poles on a regular basis, but they don't complaint. We are a resilient people; we could weather any storm. We Filipinos can endure any suffering, especially if it is for the sake of our loved ones. We do our work religiously, come hell or high water.

In general, Filipinos are a very accommodating and friendly people, especially to westerners and Americans in particular. It is no secret that, among the colonizers of the Philippines, Americans are held in high esteem to date (maybe because of your love for freedom and heroic attitude toward defending the oppressed). Friendliness and neighborliness are positive traits, which are needed also in hospital work.

Furthermore, Filipinos have a very strong sense of gratitude. A Filipino who receives favor from anybody will be forever grateful and will do his or her best to repay the act of kindness. Thus, Filipino nurses who are hired by their employers will always wish the best for their patrons and will consider them as not just employers but also as friends. While Filipino nurses can be very professional, they can also relate in a very personal manner. They are willing to give an ear or a hand to anybody. Because of all this, they show amazing resilience and commitment to quality nursing practice. Hence, Filipino nurses must be hired by United States employers.

PART II

ESSAYS AND TESTIMONIALS

CHAPTER 5

TIME FOR COLLEGE[6]

Fresh from my carefree days in high school, I decided to take a bachelor of science in nursing (BSN) course at Ateneo de Zamboanga, a Catholic and Jesuit-based college here in Zamboanga City. After enrolling in the said college, I felt nervousness and anxiety, knowing that I had come from a public school. The transition to get fit to the course was not easy and would require a lot of adjustments on my part.

I knew that getting to know new friends, classmates, teachers, and mentors was part of my mission. And I knew that I would not be alone in the struggle to survive and remain in the course until I graduated four years from now. Though I would be experiencing college bumps, it would be a must for me to be of sound mind and body— worthy to be called a "student nurse."

Becoming proactive about fighting stress and tension

---

[6] This is a revised version of the first ever article written by the author. It was published in the *Beacon* newspaper, an official publication of Ateneo de Zamboanga in August 1986.

was important to me and entailed self-discipline. Examples of good strategies for this include enough sleep, exercising regularly, and going to Mass every Sunday with my family. As the new kid on the block, I got myself involved in the objective of making friends on campus and becoming a member in community service organizations. Such organizations, to name a few, included the *BSN Pacemaker*, a nursing newsmagazine (I would go from staff writer to literary editor), the Beacon Yearbook (I would start as staff writer and eventually become managing editor), Christian Life Community (of which active member), and *Trece* newsletter (as a guest writer).

I learned that, to be successful in my college education, I had to maintain a balance between my studies and extracurricular activities. I also learned that receiving a bad grade should be a learning process and an avenue for improvement. And the experience taught me to maintain a budget for tuition, books, uniforms, and miscellaneous fees, as well as for clothing and shopping. Above all, I learned to offer myself and my college career to the Almighty God, because *college time* was one of the greatest times of my life, and that was defined by my decisions and by my actions toward meeting my goal of becoming a registered nurse.

CHAPTER 6

THE ESSENCE OF GRADUATION[7]

(Dedicated to the graduating class of 1988)

Four years ago, you left your high school days and started your college education here in our beloved Ateneo de Zamboanga. Yet the time has come for you to leave the portals of our alma mater.

Equipped with all the knowledge, skills, and proper attitudes, you are now ready to face another chapter in your life—the outside world where you will make your future through new beginnings and apply in reality what have you learned from your teachers and mentors.

You are now on your own, without your teachers on your side to prop you up. Your graduation signifies another milestone in your career. It can be life changing from a simple ceremony to an entry into your workforce.

With tears in your eyes and sadness in your hearts, you

---

[7] Original published in *Pacemaker Nursing Magazine,* the official publication of the Ateneo de Zamboanga College of Nursing, March 1988.

17

will remember your past accomplishments—good grades, honors, and the positive experiences you had all through your college life. Not to forget, if course, you'll have the memories you will keep in your heart forever.

In parting, the true essence of your graduation means you are entering into the real world and unsure what the future may bring for you. But one thing is for certain—through your fighting spirit, hard work, and perseverance, you will be able to make a difference in people's lives and in your workplace to be.

CHAPTER 7

ST. IGNATIUS AND THE PRESENT-DAY ATENEAN[8]

Dearest Lord, teach me to be generous,
to toil, and not to seek for rest.
Teach me to serve you as you deserve,
to labor, and ask not for reward,
To give and not to count the cost,
save that of knowing that I do
To fight and not to heed the wounds,
your most holy will.

If St. Ignatius of Loyola, the founder of the Society of Jesus and the patron saint of our beloved alma mater, were alive today, he would be impressed and proud of our achievements as Atenean.

In a nutshell, we've spread our wings and have flown

---

[8] Original won second-place (silver medal) in the On Spot Essay Writing Contest and was published in the *Ateneo de Zamboanga College Newsletter*, August 1989.

to the horizon to fulfill the mission and vision of our profession. In part, we do it Pro Deo et Patria (For God and Country), as our school motto states.

Imbued by the *spiritual exercises* of St. Ignatius, we strived hard to be spiritually nourished in our own selves. And we did this thanks to our Jesuit brothers and priests and lay teachers, who provided the tools that we need. Those tools included Masses, prayers, recollections, and retreats, along with the religious organizations we are in touch with, like the Christian Life Community, the Liturgical Society, Ateneo Cathetical Instruction League, and Self Actualization for Leadership Training.

We may not be the perfect Atenean as others expect us to be, but we learned one important lesson in life, and that is to counter *apathy*. Thus, our involvement in our school activities—whether its academic, community, religious, or extracurricular—and in our city's political force is absolute proofs that we are indeed men and women for others.

Moreover, our alumni graduates take pride in bringing honor in the name of our school. They do so by striving to be successful in their own respective endeavors—be they physicians, nurses, lawyers, accountants, businessmen, or whatever else.

Hence, the ideals and inspirations we learned from St. Ignatius and our Jesuit-based school led us to live life to the fullest by *example.* Our examples taught us to be role models to others; to help people to the best of our knowledge and skills through community service; and to do our utmost to be closer to and more deserving of God through prayers, gratitude, and praises.

Ad majorem Dei gloriam (for the greater glory of God).

CHAPTER 8

SUMMER ODYSSEY[9]

Summer vacation is around the corner. From the months of March to June, it is the longest break in the calendar year. This coincides with our country's tropical dry season, which lasts from March to May.

For college and universities, this break is the opportunity to offer summer classes for students who want to take advanced subjects for the next school year. Other students have the opportunity to make up time and classes by passing their failed subjects or prerequisites before the next school year begins.

So to speak, the summer vacation is a time for family *bonding*. It's a time when parents are free from the busyness of their work, and the children are free from schoolwork. This means rest and relaxation, spending quality time with loved ones, and enjoying the summer heat anywhere in our country. Of course, such activities require a sustainable budget, one that includes transportation expenses.

We can't forget that, for employers and employees,

---

[9] Original published in *AFPMC Newsletter*, June 2004.

the summer adventure is a time for a break from work. Activities like community and team building activities, including games, aim to foster camaraderie, cooperation, and unity among colleagues and coworkers outside the workplace.

In the end, the Summer Odyssey brings a variety of opportunities for us to be at our best. Bear in mind that, whatever we do or plan for the adventure getaway, safety and security is our primordial priority for everyone. And we always pray for God to guide us in our desired destination.

CHAPTER 9

COLORFUL AND MEANINGFUL[10]

I have been working in a long-term care and hospice facility for more than a year, and the most important thing I've discovered is how much I can learn from our residents.

The residents are really nice and pleasant, although some of them are confused due to Alzheimer's disease or dementia. Some of the residents are in hospice for having terminal illness, such as cancer, COPD, and the like.

What really strikes me is their patience and acceptance as they make life in a nursing facility—their second home sweet home.

In fact, such learning has inculcated in my mind and heart. As a health care provider, I have to give my best to make their lives colorful and meaningful during their stay in the facility.

Often times, a resident has really touched my heart. When he or she dies, I even go to the point of shedding

---

[10] Original available online at www.advanceweb.com in the *Tell Us Your Nursing Story Archives,* April 14, 2008, and published in the *PNANE Focus Newsletter,* December 2008.

tears with their surviving family members. I pray for them and their families, particularly during the difficult times of their lives when they have to make important decisions regarding their health.

Hence, the true essence of learning from the residents' life experiences is that it has helped me to be like their brother or friend. I am always there to help them; to listen to their stories, and to let them know that someone like me, a Filipino nurse, cares for them—no matter what the situation is.

CHAPTER 10

THE EFFECTS OF PRAYERS IN OUR LIVES[11]

May and I have been married for over ten faithful years. We've lived a happy life because we put Christ in the center of our family. Through the power of prayers, we are closer to each other and to God. Prayer also increases our faith in Him. Despite the inevitable problems and trials that have come our way, prayer always does the trick. We are enlightened, and we are committed all the more to weathering any storm. Of course, problems may not be totally eradicated, but through the power of prayer, our paradigm shifts to a better and more positive note. Thus, thanksgiving, contemplation, adoration, and supplication have been part and parcel of our family schedule.

Concrete proof of the power of prayer occurred when our daughter, Krysha May, was yet a toddler. There were instances when she would have sudden convulsions or seizures at nighttime. Medication and proper nutrition seemed not to work, so we turned to God for help. And

---

[11] Original published in the *PNANE Newsletter,* December 2008.

miracle of miracles, our daughter's predicament totally disappeared, and she grew up physically and mentally healthy.

Moreover, before coming to this great nation, we almost gave up our plan to immigrate because of the many requirements and documents that we had to accomplish before the US embassy in the Philippines. The only thing that cemented our resolve was prayer.

Our few months here in Springfield, Massachusetts, were not a walk in the park either. We had to start from scratch—no home of our own, no car, and no job security, since I still needed to take and pass the state licensure examination to become a registered nurse. Again, because of prayer and our strong faith in God, I hurdled the exams and passed with flying colors.

Sometimes we would even say to ourselves that, when God showered his blessings, our family must have been sun bathing. For today, not only did we have our own humble abode and a vehicle, but both of us also have jobs.

In conclusion, we could say that faith and prayer can really move mountains, and a real Christian should not doubt God's *love* and providence, even if it takes years before he or she experiences His goodness. God will give what we ask for, in His own time. Even before we prostrate ourselves before His altar, He already knows what we need and what's good for us. And even if He seems to be far away, we only have to trust the prophet Isaiah's words, which say, "He will never leave us orphaned." We only have to knock, and His door will be opened. We only have to ask, and we will only receive.

Actually, we don't have to look far and wide for His blessings. The air we breathe, the land we tread on, the light that emits from the sun and the moon, and our very existence are all concrete proof of God's love. Ironically, we at times even fail to thank Him for all these because they are free.

CHAPTER 11

ABOVE AND BEYOND THE CALL OF DUTY[12]

It all started when I took American Airlines Flight 1179 on September 28 from Bradley International Airport in Hartford, Connecticut, to Dallas Fort Worth Airport in Texas.

I was in seat 24F near the window of the aircraft. At the beginning of the flight, everything was fine. Many of the passengers were busy watching the in-flight movies, while others were reading the morning newspaper. Still others were sleeping. The flight attendants were busy passing out beverages; I ordered a breakfast.

All of a sudden, an hour before the aircraft landed at the DFW airport, a flight attendant made an announcement. "If there is a physician, nurse, or EMT on board, we need your help with one of our passengers," she said.

At first, I thought it was a joke, but then I got out of my seat and, together with another nurse on board, went

---

[12] Original available online at www.advanceweb.com in the *Tell Us Your Nursing Story Archives,* May 5, 2010.

to the passenger, who at the time was unresponsive and pale, her nail beds cyanotic.

Based on my assessment, I felt the passenger was exhibiting signs and symptoms of hypoglycemia, stroke, or myocardial infarction. The other nurse placed oxygen on the passenger while I checked her vitals. Her blood pressure was 90/42, pulse 45, and respiration 16. I also did a carotid massage and chest massage on the passenger.

Ultimately, as she revived, we gave the passenger (now our patient) several glasses of orange juice and ice chips. We also interviewed her husband about his wife's health history. He told us she had a history of high cholesterol and triglycerides levels, and she was taking medications and following a diet regimen for the conditions.

After several minutes, the passenger became increasingly responsive, and her condition stabilized. The only thing she remembered was that she had not eaten much for breakfast that day.

The other nurse and I implored her husband to ensure she be seen by a physician in the DFW Airport area before taking her next flight to San Francisco.

I believe we nurses need to get out of our comfort zones by helping others not just in health care facilities but in all situations, wherever we are. In doing so, we go above and beyond the call of duty.

CHAPTER 12

CHRISTIAN AWARENESS

Then Jesus said to his disciples, Whoever wishes to
come after me must deny himself, take up his cross, and
follow me. For whoever wishes to save his life will lose
it, but whoever loses his life for my sake will find it.
—Matthew 16: 24–25

My journey started in the 1989/1990 school year, when I
applied for the Jesuit Volunteers Philippines. At the time,
I was a senior student in a four-year bachelor's of science
nursing course at a Catholic and Jesuit university, were I
would soon graduate. At first, I was conditionally accepted
into the program, due to my speech problems. My faith,
courage, and determination had been tested by God before,
and another test came while I was undergoing a series of
psychological interviews by the Jesuit priests. Unknown to
myself, God already had a great plan in store for me. One
month after my graduation and while studying/reviewing
for my nurse licensure examination, I received the good
news that I had been accepted into the program.

In June of the same year, I was sent to work as

a volunteer parish nutrition worker in a fifth-class municipality province in the Visayas region specifically Sulat, Eastern Samar. I was away from the comfort of city life; away from my wants, vices, and caprices; and away from my family. For ten months, I gave my life to God and to the people with whom I dealt and worked. I conducted mothers' classes on health ·education; gave recollection to high school students; taught catechism to elementary students; and fed the poor and their families, making home visitations to those who were living lives of extreme poverty. These were the primary activities for me and my partner, Maripaz. God really prepared me for this kind of life. It was during this volunteer year that I got the chance to know my future wife, two brothers-in-law, and parents-in-law.

After my term as a volunteer, I became a full-fledged registered nurse. So I when to Metro Manila, got my license, and embarked on a six-month job hunt. During this search, May and I were already dating and in a relationship. Again, God tested my faith. After being jobless for six months, I got a stable job as a nurse in a government hospital beginning November 1991 and lasting through December 2005 before I was to go to the United States.

In the meantime, I split up with my girlfriend because I felt I was not ready to commit myself to a serious relationship with her. Besides, my priority was my career goal to come to America. It was a terribly painful situation for both of us, but we remained friends despite the breakup and continued communicating through letters and phone calls.

During this period, we both went to postgraduate school in a public and private university. She was a candidate for a master's degree in management, and I earned a master's of arts in nursing. During that time, too, she was already working as a bank teller in the province. I had a second job as a part-time assistant professor in a nursing school. In that capacity, I taught fundamentals of nursing subjects to second-year students and followed up on their clinical rotations, both in the hospital and community.

***

Rejoice always. Pray without ceasing. In all circumstances give thanks, for this is the will of God for you in Christ Jesus.
—1 Thessalonians 5:16–18

God really works in mysterious ways. While my girlfriend and I were broken up, her parents and two brothers, who were both priests, continued to pray that somehow and someday the two of us would be back in each other's arms. True enough and through the power of prayer, two years later, I felt those flickering feelings that told me I was meant for her. So in April 25, 1998, we got married. Nine months later, our bundle of joy baby girl, Krysha May, was born. Those were the happiest moments we'd had in our lives. Our first few years of our married life had been a mixture of misunderstandings, word wars, and lovers' quarrels. Yet through prayers, thanksgiving, and praise, we were able to patch things up and make ends meet.

Our family relationship with God and the Holy Trinity was further deepened when my sister introduced us to the Divine Mercy prayers, novena, and rosary. We surrendered everything to God. From time to time, we did our pilgrimages to the National Shrine of the Divine Mercy, only miles from where we live.

In addition, at that time, I resumed my plans for myself and my family to seek greener pastures in the United States. After taking, failing, and passing those English and nursing examinations so many times, I was finally rewarded. God has been good to me and my family. How? After ten years of waiting, finally our dreams came true.

However, before coming to this great nation, we almost gave up our plan to emigrate because of the many requirements and documents we had to accomplish and complete for the US embassy in the Philippines.

Finally, in 2006 we landed in Springfield, Massachusetts.

Our first few months here in this nation were no a walk in the park either. We had to start from scratch. We had no home of our own, no car, and no job security, since I still needed to take and pass the state licensure examination to become a registered nurse.

Because of our strong faith in God, I hurdled the exams with flying colors. In addition, our daughter was an outstanding student in English and reading at her elementary school.

After passing the said state licensure examination, I worked at Genesis HealthCare in the Heritage Hall West and Heritage Hall North facilities for two years, first for a contract year and then for a year as a regular nurse. I was filled with gratitude to God for bringing me and my family to this land of milk and honey. My wife had her share of reward too because she got a job in the same facility where I was working.

Moreover, I discovered that God's gift to me as a freelance writer was further developed—or shall I say *harnessed.* Although I had already started writing while back in the Philippines before moving to this beautiful country (I'd been doing so since 2006), new developments in this arena manifested here. Several of my articles were published, both in print and on the web, in leading local and national nursing journals, magazines, and newsletters here in this country. Some of the publications even paid me for a job well done and for inspiring other nurses to make a difference in their patients' lives.

Meanwhile, my wife and I were actively involved with the Knights of Columbus council and their spouses. Our daughter was involved in the weekend Catholic Catechism Development program of the Our Lady of Mount Carmel Church. Likewise, we continued our pilgrimages to the National Shrine of the Divine Mercy in Stockbridge. Our involvement has deepened not only our faith but also our "Christian awareness" about the importance of being of service and being role models to our fellow men, as well as to the community and church with which we are connected.

On the other hand, on Labor Day, September 1, 2008, what could have been our second child did not materialize. My wife had a miscarriage on that fateful day. We were so depressed and devastated about losing our second child to be. Yet we never blamed ourselves. Nor did we blame God. We know there are reasons why such things have to happen. In fact, we became closer to each other and to God. In addition, our faith in Him increased. All the more, we are enlightened and are committed to weathering any storm because He always does the trick.

***

Trust in the Lord with all thine heart; and
lean not unto thine own understanding.
—Proverbs 3:5

In October 2009, we moved to McKinney, Texas, not knowing that God had prepared something for us. I was fortunate to land a job at the Medical Center of Plano, and my wife landed one at a rehabilitation center. God is good all the time, and all the time He is good. After three months of working in the hospital, I end up working at the same facility where my wife was working. It was as if God was telling me, "You should work together with your wife, to make a better team."

As usual, my family and I were actively involved with the Knights of Columbus and with other programs and activities, this time around at St. Gabriel the Archangel Catholic Community (SGACC).

When Father Don Zeiler, the pastor at SGACC, announced at one of the Sunday Masses he officiated that there would be an incoming Christ Renews His Parish (CRHP) renewal weekend for men and women, my wife and I felt that flickering feeling, telling us the Holy Spirit was inviting us to experience God's full presence. We were supported by our families on both sides as we prepared to partake in this one-of-a-kind adventure of a lifetime. At first, the reason we wanted to participate in such an activity was to renew our faith. But God gave us many surprises, adding much to our expectations.

With full trust in Him, and with the CRHP XVI staff who conducted the said weekend, we attended the renewal weekend. The experiences we had with the Lord in the renewal process were marvelous. We were able to develop a good personal relationship with Him, admitting and confessing to our sins and accepting that we are humans, subject to sins, errors, and mistakes.

Life following the CRHP renewal weekend has never been the same again for my wife and me. It was as if God was telling us, "I, your Lord and teacher, have just washed your feet. You, then, should wash one another's feet." Yes, we still have periods of ups and downs in our family relationship. But with the many spiritual lessons we've learned from CRHP—coupled with prayers, putting Christ as the center of our family, and using the Holy Family as our model to emulate—we are able to make things better.

As a token of thankfulness and gratefulness, my family and I additionally became involved with the Men's Club and CRHP. This is our way of sharing our talents and time and giving back to our fellow parishioners for all the blessings and graces God has given us.

***

Be on your guard; stand firm in the faith;
be men of courage; be strong. Your every
act should be done with love.
—1 Corinthians 16:13–14

***

Though I resigned from my job in November 2011, God had led the way for a better workplace for me. After a month, I was hired at Plano Specialty Hospital. True to God's promise, I found a family in my new employers, where peace, harmony, unity, camaraderie, support, and help are present among staff. In addition, patients and their families are good and kind, though at times they can be rude and arrogant—which is normal for us in the health care system.

Hence, we truly believe that faith and prayer can move mountains. And a real Christian should not doubt God's love and providence at all times, even if it takes years before he or she experiences His goodness. God will give what we ask for, in His own time.

The author, a third-degree knight of the Knights of Columbus council and a member of the Men's Club, shared this witness story to the thirteen participants of the St. Gabriel the Archangel Catholic community's Christ Renews His Parish (CRHP) Batch XVIII for Men Renewal Weekend, May 19–20, 2012. The author and his wife attended CRHP XVII in October 2011 and, since then, continuously experience the changes and transformations that God and the Holy Spirit work in their lives as one happy family.

CHAPTER 13

A DECADE OF AMERICAN FRIENDSHIP[13]

The long journey of coming to the United States of America started when I crossed the hurdle of passing the Commission on Graduates of Foreign Nursing Schools (CGFNS) qualifying examination back in January 1995. From that time on, mine and my family's pain, struggle, and trials began and eventually ended when we arrived in the nation popularly known as the "land of milk and honey."

Having applied to some recruitment agencies in 1995, 2000, and 2002, and having passed the TOEFL (Test of English as a Foreign Language) and IELTS (International English Language Testing System) tests, I was able to satisfy the ICHP's additional requirements (aside from the CGFNS certificate) to obtain a VisaScreen certificate for an employment-based immigrant visa.

God marvelously worked in mysterious ways for our family. Just when we thought that our plan to immigrate to the United States would remain an elusive and futile

---

[13] Original available online at www.facebook.com/joeljongclemente, March 2, 2016.

dream, He came to the rescue. In November 2005, we had our interview at the US embassy in Manila. Thereafter, in the first quarter of 2006, our American dream came true when we landed in Massachusetts and New York State. Seven years later, we moved to our beautiful home state of Texas, where we finally found our niche.

Looking back, after a decade of American friendship, we are proud to say that it was worth the wait. Patience, as they say, is indeed a virtue. For even during our anxiety, God was gracious. We were privileged to witness the ordination to the priesthood of my two brothers-in-law and attended a number of family reunions prior to our departure to this great nation.

For the blessings we received, we are thankful to our parents, brothers, sisters, relatives, friends, the Horizon Recruitment Pacific Corporation, Worldwide HealthStaff Ltd., and the Genesis HealthCare Corporation. But most of all we are grateful for the divine providence without which good things would be entirely impossible. As payback, we try to make a difference in other people's lives, specifically through our commitment and dedication in caring for our patients. In our own little way, we also try to build a better world through community service, supporting community projects and church fundraisers for our less privileged brethren and victims of calamities, and even joining prayer vigils to make this world a better place to live in.

Indeed, God listens to those who call, opens the door for those who knock, and grants seekers what they look for. We just need to persistently cling to Him, and everything will be given us. We should not doubt His love and providence, even if it takes years before we experience His goodness.

CHAPTER 14

KRYSHA MAY AT EIGHTEEN: HER DAD'S UNSOLICITED DISCLOSURE[14]

Eighteen years ago, our lovely, cute, and cuddly baby girl was born at AFP Medical Center in Quezon City, Philippines. We, her parents, as well as her grandparents and uncles, were and are truly proud, blessed, and thankful to have her as our bundle of joy. She is the only grandchild from our Cabuenas family.

While other only children end up being spoiled brats or black sheep in their families, Krysha May was the exact opposite. She grew up to be a kindhearted, generous, good, and loving daughter to us; grandchild to her *lolo* and *lola* (grandpa and grandma); niece to her uncles and aunties; and friend to her cousins, classmates, and circle of friends.

Just like a normal child, she had her share of childhood illness, such as measles. We were in and out of the hospital

---

[14] Original available online at www.facbook.com/kryshaclemente, January 29, 2017.

for the said predicament. Yet with prayers, faith and trust in God, she grew up to be physically and mentally healthy.

Being raised in a very Catholic community, she subsequently changed her outlook on life from one that was care free to one that rendered her a law abiding and God-fearing child. This is not surprising, as both her grandparents are actively involved in the church, her two uncles are diocesan priests, and we her parents are devotees of the Divine Mercy.

Who would have thought that, at four, Krysha May would became a "Little Queen" in her own right? She won the titles "Little Queen Kaypian" and "Miss United Nation 1st runner-up." In addition, she bagged the "Best in Talent and Best Float" award attesting to her beauty and brain prowess. Such competitions took place way back in 2003 in our Barangay community and in the prekindergarten school she attended.

At the age of seven, Krysha May and we, her parents, successfully migrated to the United States of America. While it is true that the move was the fulfillment of our American dream, it was not an easy transition for her. It was not easy to face the new life she would be embracing in a foreign land. But as the saying goes, *"Life must go on."* Krysha May eventually was able to adjust to the way of life, climate, and culture of our second home sweet home in the United States.

While she was in first and third grade at Daniel Brunton Elementary School and White Street School (WSS), both in Springfield, Massachusetts (MA), she was consistently the highest achiever in English and reading. For this, she was honored by the state, receiving the MA MassMutual Outstanding Achievement award for three consecutive years. She was also the recipient of the Outstanding Academic Performance in English/Language Arts District Assessments for the 2008–2009 school year at WSS. Her testimonial story regarding her journey from the Philippines to this great nation was simultaneously published and posted at the WSS news and literary bulletin board in the same school year.

Her claim to this small fame continued during her fourth and fifth grade years at Mooneyham Elementary School in McKinney, Texas. She was awarded the Texas Assessment of Knowledge and Skills (TAKS) Academic Medal award for two years in English and reading (2009–2011). She also garnered "advanced high" in the Texas English Language Proficiency Assessment System (TELPAS) while studying at the aforementioned school, again for two years.

Krysha May's proficiency in English and reading continued to score her touchdowns while she was enrolled at Sam and Ann Roach Middle School. There, she was a recipient of the "Good Writer and Excellence" award for writing excellence. She also bagged the "Music Excellence" award for piano at the Music Institute of North Texas for two years while in middle school (2013 and 2014).

Her stint in high school started in 2014 and continues as of this writing at Heritage High School (HHS) in Frisco, Texas. She has proven herself to be a "youth for others" Pro Deo et Patria (for God and Country)—as evidenced by her social awareness and involvement in both community and service organizations. Specifically, she is involved in the Philanthropy Club at HHS and the Youth Club at St. Gabriel the Archangel Catholic community. Sharing her talent, skills, and time by volunteering to help bring about events like the annual Jesse's Tree gift-giving ceremony for Christmas, pancake breakfasts, spaghetti dinners, and the Frisco Fun Run has been an important part of her transformation into a service-oriented youth. And these contributions are also concrete proof of her caring attributes; she cares for people and for the community in general. She has clearly inherited the traits of her father, grandfather, and two uncles, who are men for others.

Meanwhile, on the lighter side, Krysha May continues to play the piano and goes to her college preparatory school during the weekend.

As she celebrates her eighteenth birthday today (January 29), we—her dad and mom, grandparents, uncles, and relatives—wish her more blessings and grace, good health, and fulfillment of her dreams. May she always be grateful and thankful for and contented with what she has in life. May she continue to offer praise and thanksgiving to the author of all that is good and the provider of all that we need. May she learn how to pay it forward, especially to our less privileged brethren.

May she not forget where she comes from, especially our Filipino values and good traits, as they are guiding principles and foolproof recipes for success. And may she always be safe on the road as she now drives her favorite toy—her car.

God bless you, our dear Krysha! Know that we always love you and are here always here for you!

PART III

FEATURES

CHAPTER 15

I AM A CRITICAL CARE NURSE[15]

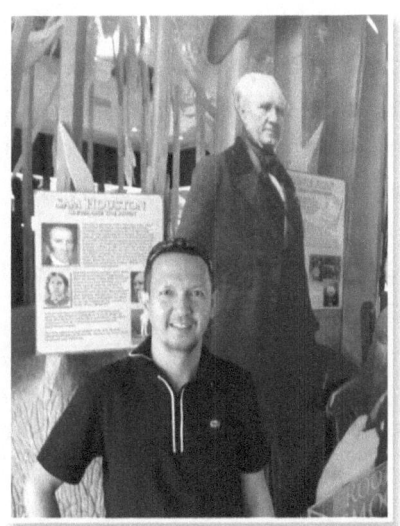

Joel J. Clemente, RN, MAN, is a staff nurse in the critical care unit at Plano Specialty Hospital in Plano, Texas.

[15] Copyright 2014, American Association of Critical-Care Nurses doi: http://dxdoi.org/10.4037/ccn2014660. Clemente, JJ. I Am a Critical Care Nurse. *Crit Care Nurse* 2014 34(2): 84. All rights reserved. Reprinted with permission from AACN.

Why did you become a nurse?

I want to help people reach their optimum level of functioning. Respect, compassion, dedication to work, and love for God have been my cornerstone as a nurse. Being a nurse has fulfilled the American dream for me and my family after years of struggle and hardship.

What about your job as a nurse makes you happy?

Seeing patients recover slowly but surely and knowing I was part of that recovery gives me a sense of joy. Also, it is meaningful when patients die with dignity and peace, with their families supporting them. The warm camaraderie, unity, and support I enjoy with my coworkers mean much to me as well. All in all, being a critical care nurse is a blessing because I am able to develop the knowledge, skills, and attitudes I want in my daily life.

Tell us about an extraordinary experience you've had as a critical care nurse.

A few years ago I was on an American Airlines flight when the crew announced that they needed a doctor or nurse because a passenger was having a health problem. Together with another nurse, I gave first aid treatment to the passenger, who was experiencing severe hypoglycemia episodes. We gave her orange juice, crackers, and a carotid massage, then took her vital signs. After a few minutes, the passenger's condition stabilized. This situation taught me that helping people get back on their feet and be healthy not only applies in health care facilities but in everyday life as well.

What are the challenges you encounter and how do you overcome them?

My major challenge, which is personal, is not fully trusting myself. Every day, I try to overcome it by praying to God, asking questions, and seeking advice from my family and coworkers.

What has your journey as a nurse been like?

My journey has led me to discover so many new things along the way, like high-tech equipment, materials, and procedures; electronic medical records; new friends; and breakthroughs affecting the health care delivery system— all for the betterment of patients and their families.

At the end of a busy day, how do you find balance in your life?

I find balance being with my spouse and our child. We pray, attend church, watch television, and do things around the house together, all of which strengthen our family relationship. We prioritize quality time together despite our busy schedules, and adhere to our motto, "The family that prays together, stays together." It is important to be able to relieve my stress and tension from work because, before I can take care of my patients, I need to be strong and healthy, physically and emotionally.

What would we be surprised to know about you?

I come across as a serious person, but really I am a cheerful guy and I like to joke around, especially to lighten up stressful times. Also, despite my hectic schedule with both family and work, I am still able to make a difference and help build a better world through community service and prayers as a member of the Knights of Columbus Council and Men's Club at St. Gabriel the Archangel Catholic Community.

How has AACN played a role in your career?

AACN has given me the tools I need to be an exceptional critical care nurse. I take the free CNE tests, and the journals keep me informed of the latest news, trends, and research in critical care nursing. AACN is offering review materials I need to prepare for the Adult CCRN certification examination. AACN has been a resource for both personal and professional goals.

("I Am a Critical Care Nurse" features the extraordinary in a critical care nurse's ordinary experiences. To be featured in this department, contact Critical Care Nurse *via e-mail at ccn@aacn.org.)*

PART IV

CLASS HISTORY

CHAPTER 16

PLEXUS '90: A CARAVAN OF PROFESSIONALS

Fresh from their carefree days in high school, in June 1986, more than three hundred students started their career as future prudent nurses in the Nursing Division of the Ateneo de Zamboanga college community. Though puerile and unseasoned, they embraced the challenge to journey over the road less traveled and to discover the world of nursing education, practice, and research.

In December of the same year, while still in their freshmen status, this vibrant caravan made history in the entire Ateneo campus by winning the first overall championship ever in the school's annual sports festival—a gargantuan lift for the Nursing Division since its 1980 pioneer graduates.

Eventually, these student nurses had their cap badge ceremony at the school's Sacred Heart Chapel in November 1987. Overcoming the major hurdles of passing the basic fundamentals of nursing, along with anatomy and physiology and microbiology and parasitology with flying colors was, indeed, a true and lasting accomplishment.

During their junior year, the 1988/1989 school year, the aforementioned students tackled the challenges of having to experience a more complex and difficult area of nursing in the medical-surgical specialty. Some also experienced financial difficulty. Yet with courage and determination, coupled with prayers and faith in God, they moved to the next level of their academic pursuit. On the lighter side, they had their memorable Junior-Senior Prom with their predecessor—Phoenix Class '89.

Their senior year, 1989/1990, was the year where they chose "Plexus '90," a.k.a. "networks," as their class name. In December, the students witnessed the giving of the Hall of Fame awards to the Nursing Division from the entire Ateneo community for being the overall champions in the school sports fest from 1986 to 1989. Likewise, they won first place in the annual Christmas choral festival this time, after landing second place for three consecutive years (from 1986 through 1988).

Despite their busy schedules both in the classroom and in the clinical areas, the group was also actively involved in other school programs. This included the BSN Acquaintance Party, Christmas Love Drive, Choral and Sports festival, Christian Life Community, Muslim Student Association, Social Awareness for Community Service Involvement, Writers' Club, Self Actualization for Leadership Training, the senior retreat, the Medical-Dental Mission, and a lot more. All of this was a concrete testament that this group of young bloods embodied the Ateneo mission of Pro Deo et Patria.

Finally, in March 1990, these 140 dedicated men and

women (including others who belonged to the eleventh batch of BSN graduates and who also belonged to the third batch of the Revised BSN Curriculum) officially graduated from the Ateneo de Zamboanga College of Nursing. In part, they had their exclusive nursing graduation in a pin and ring ceremony, where some of them were recipients of the Clinical Efficiency awards, receiving Community Service, Perfect Attendance, and Player Certificate titles.

Although everyone has gone their separate ways to follow their dreams and the mission of their profession, these Ateneo nurses have never forgotten their class name. The networks and networking formed during those years are very much alive to date, thanks to social media. There is open communication, and everybody is updated about each other's activities and circumstances.

In December 2015, after twenty-five long years, this caravan of professional nurses gathered once more with pride and joy, not only to celebrate their silver anniversary as a group but also to reminisce about their Ateneo days and to rekindle their friendships and the bond they built. After all, having fun, getting inspired, reconnecting, launching the Scholarship Fund project of the Ateneo College of Nursing, and reaching out to their beloved Zamboanga City in the name of their class, Plexus '90, through community service and batch-sponsored activities were the foremost goals of their once-in-a-lifetime reunion.

The author, who was the class historian and representative of the Plexus '90 batch, wrote this history at the time of their twenty-fifth class homecoming alumni reunion, December 2015. Such history was also published in the Plexus '90 at 25 Souvenir Book, *December 2015.*

PART V

POETRY

THE FIRST CHRISTMAS[16]

Two thousand years ago ...
The Savior was born in a manger
Covered with swaddling clothes
With St. Joseph and the Blessed Virgin Mary ...
In the little town of Bethlehem.

While shepherds watched their flock ...
They saw a bright new light.
And from heaven above ...
A choir of angels sang *Gloria In Excelsis Deo.*

From the East came Three Wise Men ...
Who visited and paid homage to baby Jesus.
Then opening their treasure chests ...
They offered Him gifts of gold, frankincense, and myrrh.

Up to this day ...
The message of that First Christmas remains the same—
That is, to love one another as we love ourselves.

---

[16] Original published in the *AFPMC Newsletter,* December 1999.

And no matter what ...
In every corner of the world,
There will always be Christmas ...
In every human's heart and soul.

A PRUDENT NURSE[17]

A good nurse exerts extra efforts in rendering
Utmost care to her patients ...
To the best of her knowledge, skills, and
Attitude as a health care provider.

In time of her patients' sorrows and pain ...
She empathizes with their feelings and concerns,
Lending a helping hand; giving touch therapy; and
Providing psychological, emotional, and moral support.

Though being called as the physician's handmaiden
In carrying out doctors' orders ...
She always inculcates the Nightingale's
Pledge in all her undertakings,
Becoming more assertive and independent and, at all
Times, ensuring patients' safety and protection.

Whatever and whenever situations arise ...
She maintains her integrity as a professional nurse,
Thus, playing a key role in the health care delivery
System and carrying out the goals of the
Nursing profession.

---

[17] Original published in the *AFPMC Newsletter*, May 2001.

Indeed, these are the significant qualities that a
Prudent nurse truly possesses ...
Making her unique and her profession
A noble one.
And ultimately, she serves as God's instrument in
Promoting and restoring the health
Of her patients.

NOTHING LASTS FOREVER[18]

Jewelry that glitters
Is not all genuine.
Some is plated, fancy, or fake,
And does not last forever.

Beauty and fame are temporary.
In time, they lost their perfection.
Like gold, silver, and bronze
They do not last forever.

New flowers grows on trees
And bloom beautifully.
But old flowers fall and dry
Because they do not last forever.

Bad deeds are remembered for a lifetime.
Yet good deeds are not appreciated
In the long run.
They do not last forever.

---

[18] Original published in *Springfield Technical and Community College Literature Report,* April 2008.

And people of all walks of life,
Whether good or bad,
Don't last forever.
Eventually, they die, young or old.

PART VI

RECOGNITION CORNER

CHAPTER 17

HONORS AND AWARDS

From the ADZ College News

Joel Clemente was awarded a silver medal for winning second place in the On the Spot Essay Writing Contest on the theme "St. Ignatius and the Present-Day Atenean," held July 1989 at the college's Learning Resource Building. The contest was conducted in celebration of the feast of St. Ignatius of Loyola, which fell on July 31.[19]

From the ADZ CON News

Joel Clemente, together with his fellow ten batch mates, were recipients of the Community Service award for unselfishly sharing their knowledge, expertise, and utmost support in community service activities. The awarding ceremony was held March 1990 during their BSN Plexus

---

[19] *Ateneo de Zamboanga College Newsletter,* August 1989.

1990 Graduation / Pin and Ring Ceremony at the college's Sacred Heart Chapel.[20]

From the Recognition News

Joel Clemente, RN, BSN, MAN, of Heritage Hall West (MA) has recently joined the newsletter committee for the Philippine Nurses Association of New England (PNANE). As a contributing writer, Joel will submit articles on a variety of nursing topics. One of his first articles, published in February, addressed the topic "How Could Television Improve Its Portrayal of Nurses?" Joel, well done![21]

From the CHEERS

Kudos to Heritage Hall West (MA) nurse Joel Clemente, RN, BSN, MAN, who recently joined the newsletter committee for the Philippine Nurses Association of New England (PNANE). Joel is a contributing writer, submitting articles on several nursing topics. A recent article discussed "How Could Television Improve Its Portrayal of Nurses?"[22]

From a resident and an administrator

"Joel works very hard and is always a gentlemen with all the different personalities he deals with. Thanks for always being a gentleman." What a nice compliment from a resident.[23]

---

[20] *Ateneo de Zamboanga College of Nursing Flyer,* March 1990.
[21] Genesis HealthCare *Vitals Newsletter,* March 2008.
[22] Genesis HealthCare *The Big Blue Reprint,* March 10, 2008.
[23] Baybrooke Village Care & Rehab Center *Shining Star Employee Recognition,* February 24, 2010.

AFP Medical Center Commendations

Joel received ten commendations while working at AFP Medical Center from 1997 to 2004, one certificate of recognition from Concordia College (CC) and two certificates of appreciation from AFPMC Civilian Employee's Association (CEA) prior to his departure to the United States.[24]

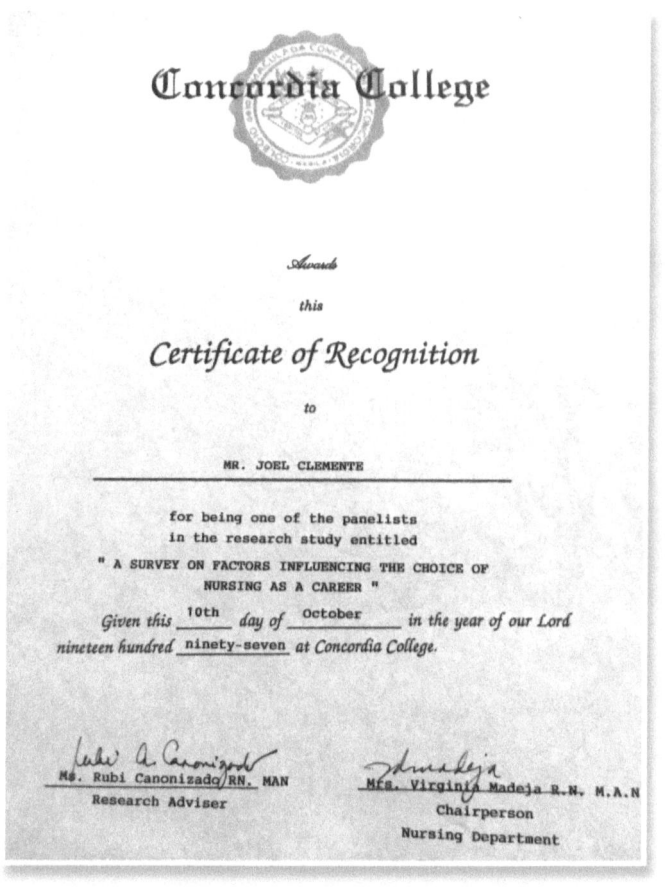

Concordia College

Awards

this

Certificate of Recognition

to

MR. JOEL CLEMENTE

for being one of the panelists
in the research study entitled

" A SURVEY ON FACTORS INFLUENCING THE CHOICE OF
NURSING AS A CAREER "

Given this 10th *day of* October *in the year of our Lord*
nineteen hundred ninety-seven *at Concordia College.*

Ms. Rubi Canonizado/RN. MAN
Research Adviser

Mrs. Virginia Madeja R.N. M.A.N
Chairperson
Nursing Department

---

[24] *AFPMC; AFPMC CEA*, March 19, 2004; *CC College of Nursing*, October 10, 1997.

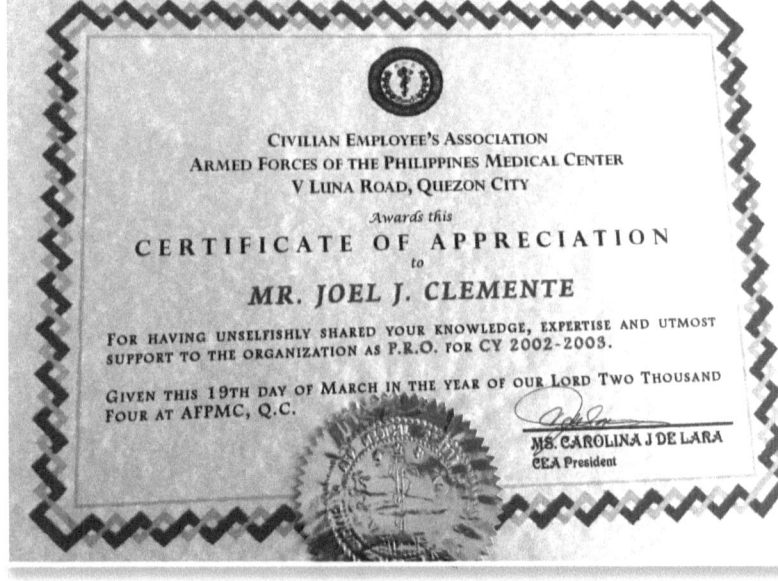

CHAPTER 18

AMERICAN AIRLINES

Executive Office
October 8, 2009

Mr. Joel Clemente
71 Wilcox Street
Springfield, MA 01105

Dear Mr. Clemente:

Please accept our company's formal "Thank You" for the assistance you provided aboard flight 1179, which operated from Hartford to Dallas, Fort Worth. We are all grateful that you were on board and freely offered your medical expertise when it was needed most. Without a doubt, you greatly improved a difficult situation on September 28.

As a tangible expression of our appreciation for volunteering your time and experience, we have enclosed a transportation voucher. The voucher is valid for one year from the date of issue. While the voucher itself is a nontransferable and cannot be sold or bartered, you may use it to buy a ticket for a friend or relative if you prefer.

Mr. Clemente, I realize your offer of assistance was not motivated by any potential reward. Nevertheless, we wanted you to know how much your efforts were appreciated – and that we look forward to serving you again soon. It will be our privilege to welcome you aboard American Airlines when your plans call for travel by air.

Sincerely,
Thomas N. Bettes, MD, MPH
Director, Medical and
Occupational Health Services

Enclosure

THE FLORENCE NIGHTINGALE PLEDGE[25]

I solemnly pledge myself before God and in the presence of this assembly to pass my life in purity and to practice my profession faithfully. I will abstain from whatever is deleterious and mischievous, and will not take or knowingly administer any harmful drug.

I will do all in my power to maintain and elevate the standard of my profession and will hold in confidence all personal matters committed to my keeping, and all family affairs coming to my knowledge in the practice of my calling.

With loyalty will I endeavor to aid the physician in his work and devote myself to the welfare of those committed to my care.

---

[25] Based on Lystra Gretter and a Committee for the Farrand Training School for Nurses in Detroit, Michigan, who created the pledge in 1893, in honor of Florence Nightingale, the founder of modern nursing.

PHOTO GALLERY

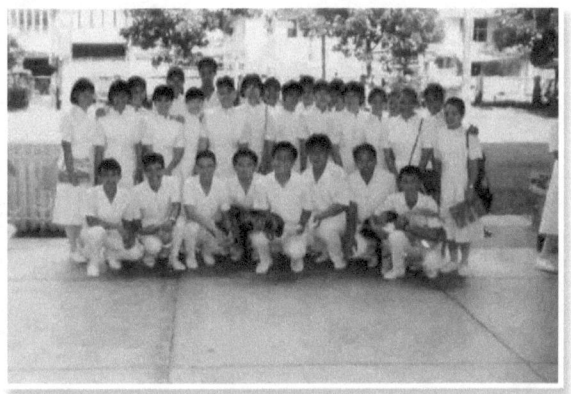

Joel's BSN college days with his fellow batchmates circa 1987

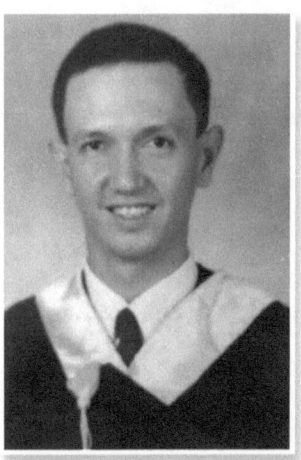

Joel's MAN post graduate photo circa April 1997

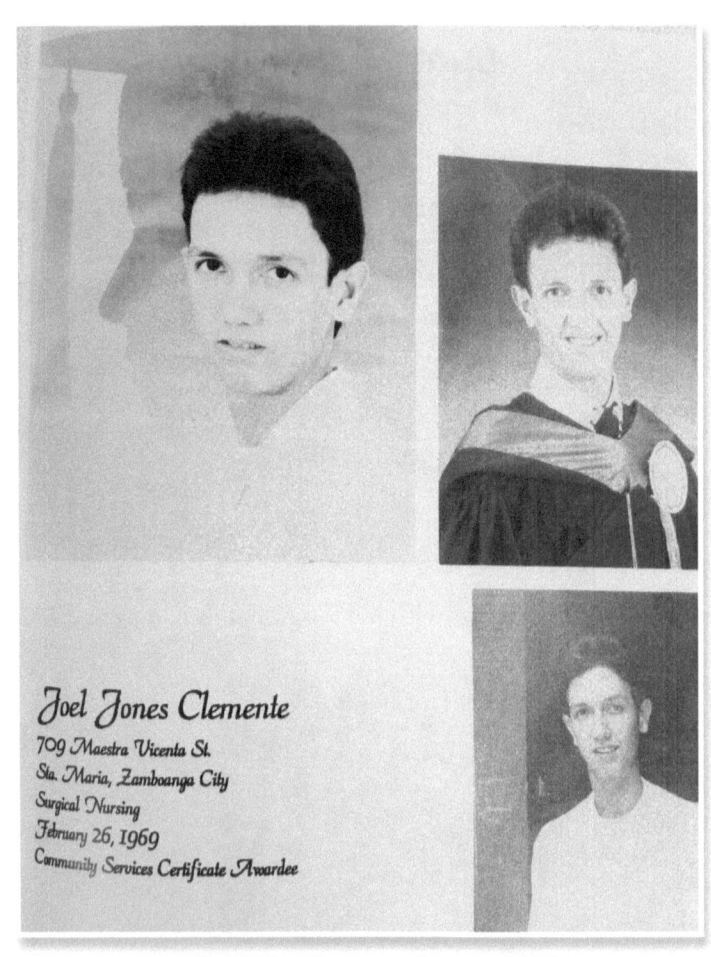

Joel Jones Clemente
709 Maestra Vicenta St.
Sta. Maria, Zamboanga City
Surgical Nursing
February 26, 1969
Community Services Certificate Awardee

Joel's BSN college graduation 1990

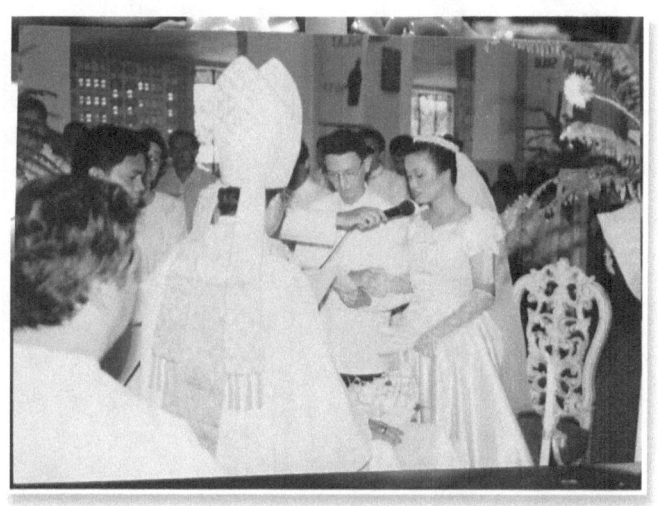

Joel & May's wedding with Bishop Leonardo Medroso,
April 25, 1998

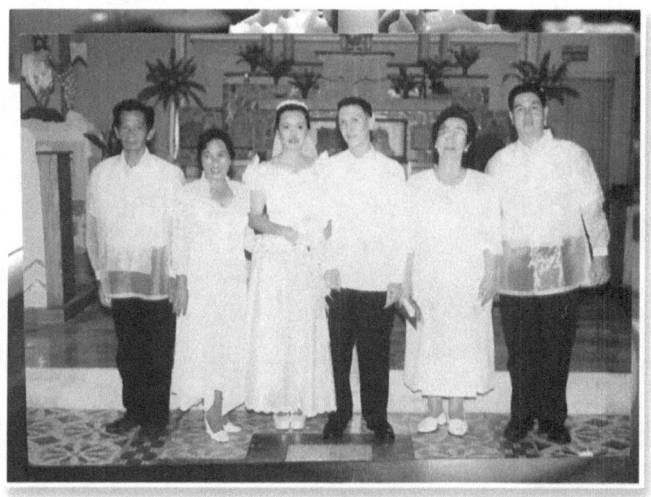

Joel & May's wedding with their parents, April 25, 1998

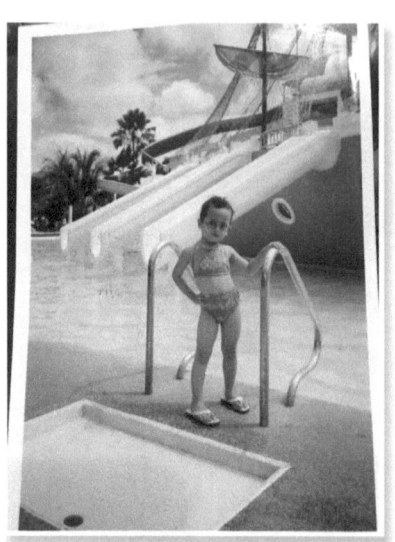

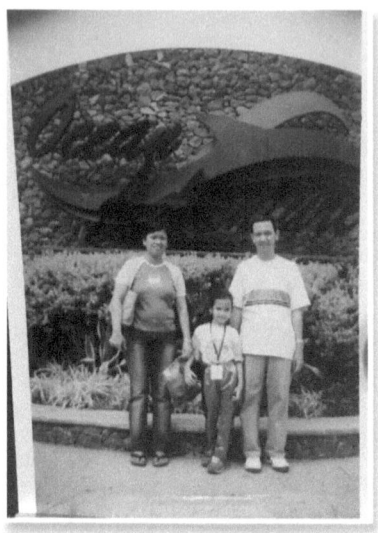

Joel & May's only
child Krysha May

The Clemente family at
Ocean Adventure

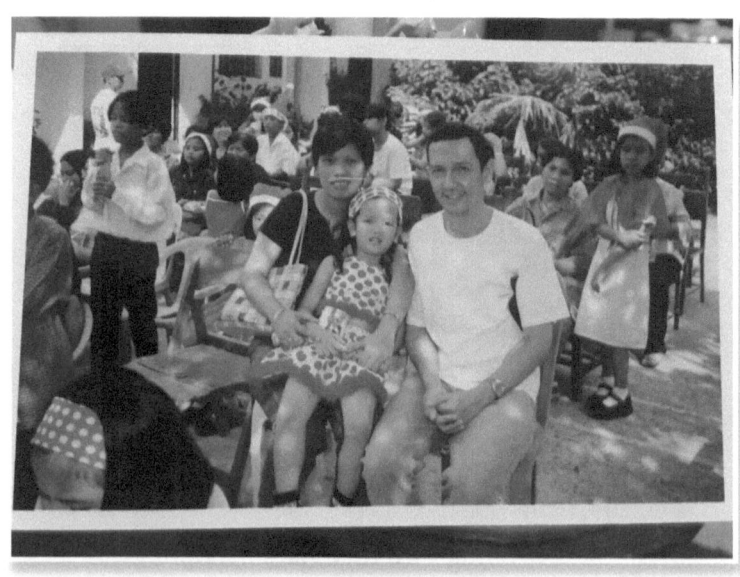

The Clemente family during their
Palmera Phase 4B days

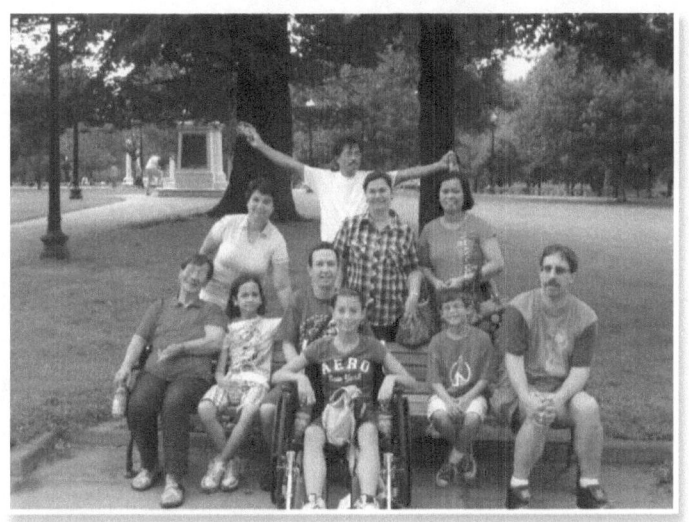

Clemente, Elopre & Yeosock family vacation
in Boston, Massachusetts

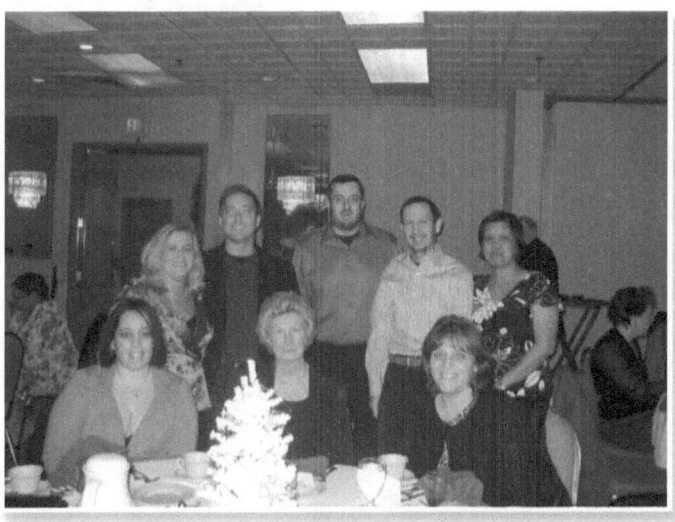

Joel & May with their fellow Heritage Hall North nursing staff

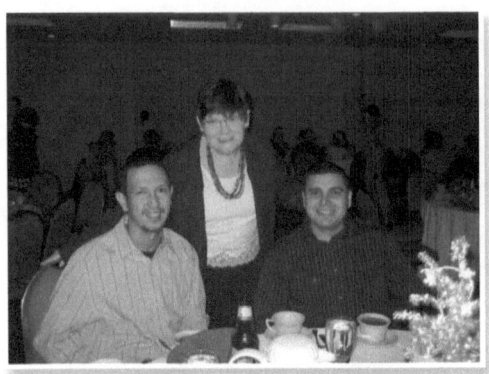

Joel with his fellow Heritage
Hall West nursing staff

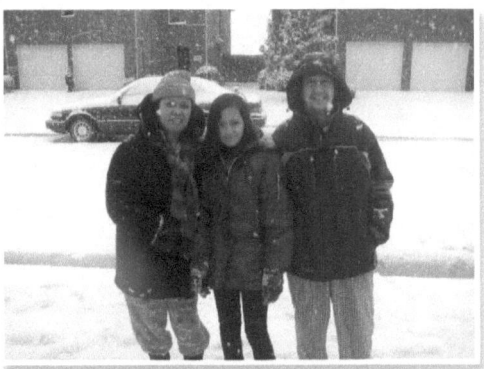

Joel & May enjoying the winter
season in North Texas

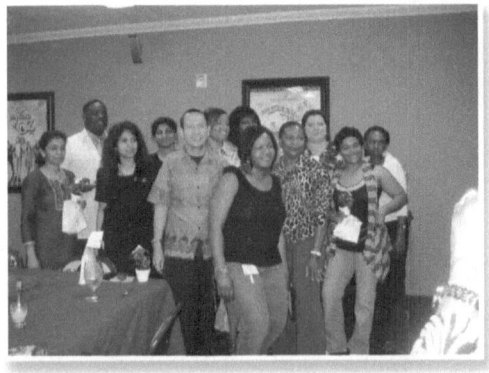

Nurses' Week celebration at Baybrooke
Village Care & Rehab Center

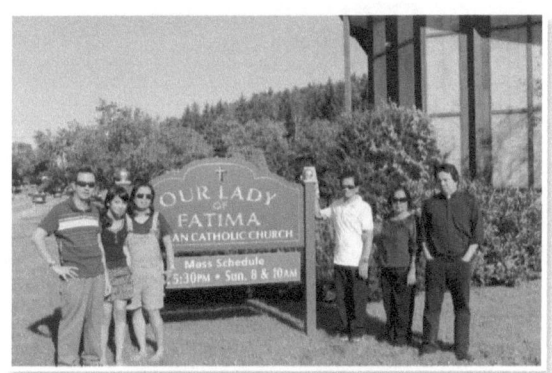

Cabuenas & Clemente family
in Wilmington, Vermont

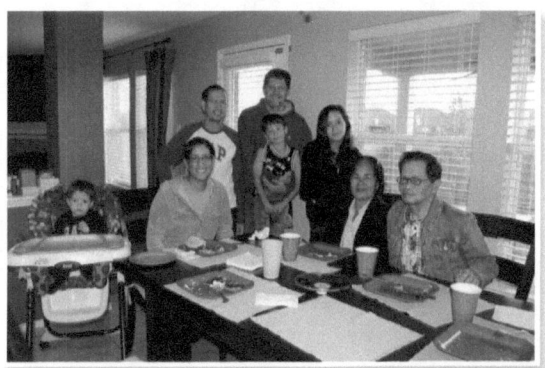

Dinner with the Oaks family

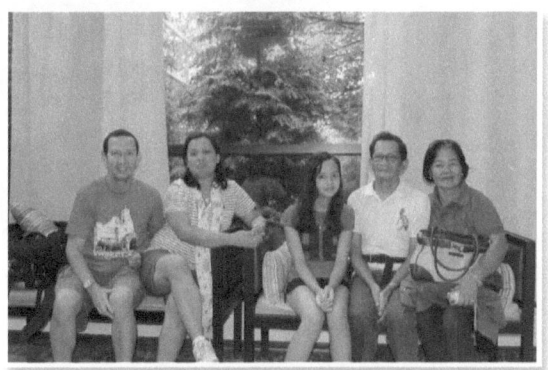

Cabuenas & Clemente
family in New York

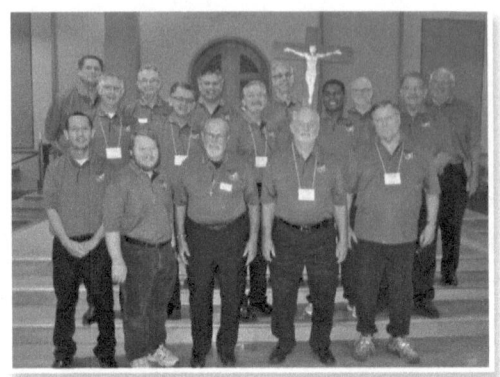

Joel with his fellow Christ Renews
His Parish (CHRP) brothers

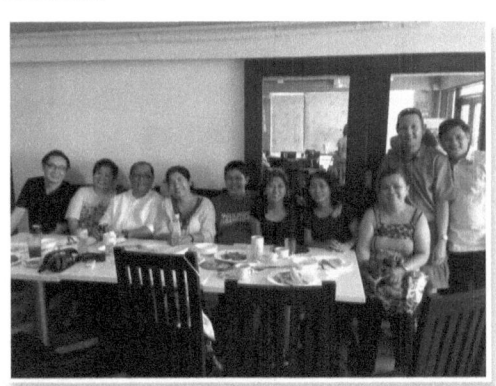

Joel with his fellow JVP 11 batchmates

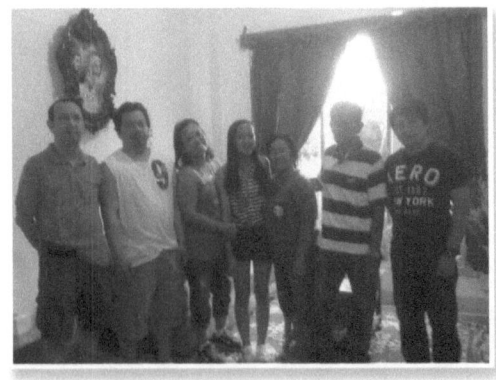

Cabuenas & Clemente's
family reunion 2013

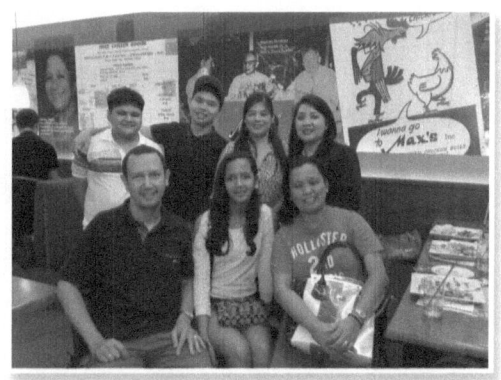

Joel with his fellow Sta. Maria
Elementary school '82 batchmates

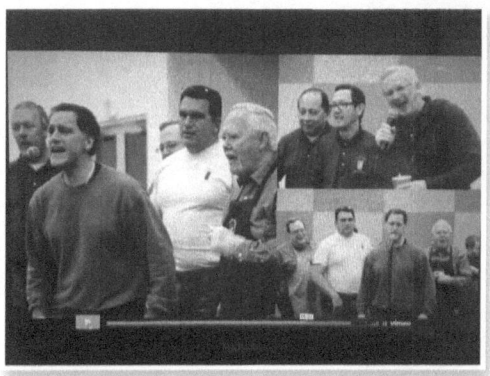

Joel with his fellow Men's Club brothers

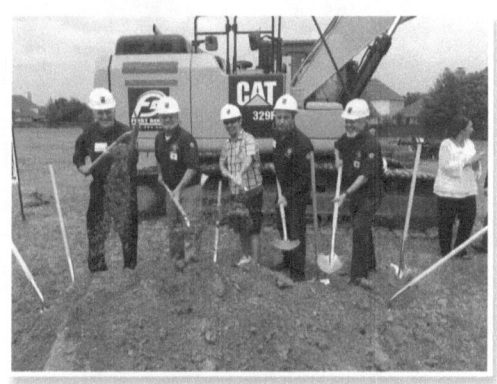

Joel with his fellow Knights
of Columbus brothers

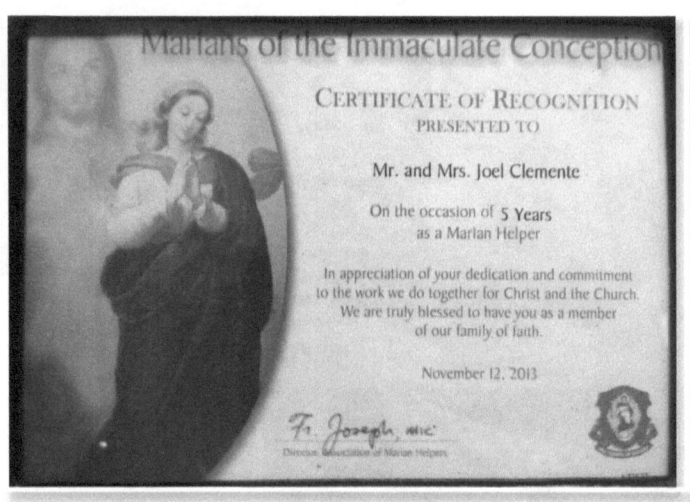

A Recognition for Joel & his wife May

Joel & May with Fr. Don Zeiler

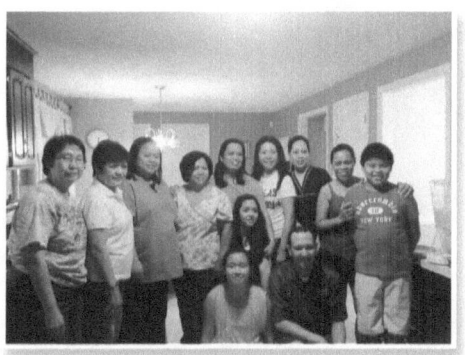

The Clemente's circle of friends
of Western Massachusetts

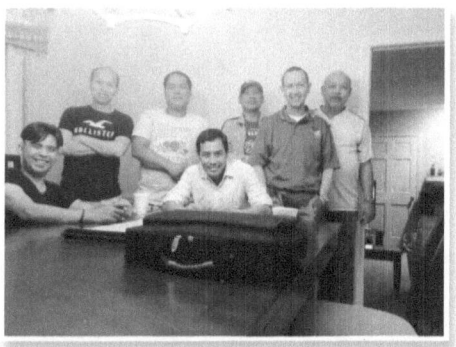

The Clemente's circle of friends
of Western Massachusetts

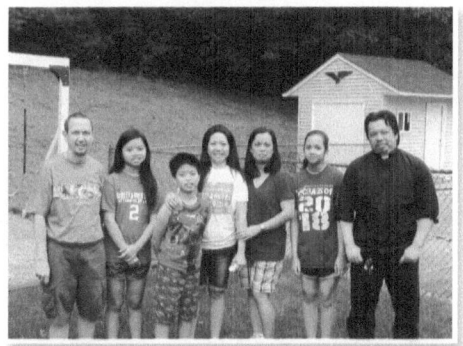

The Clemente's with the Basa
family & Fr. Cyrain Cabuenas

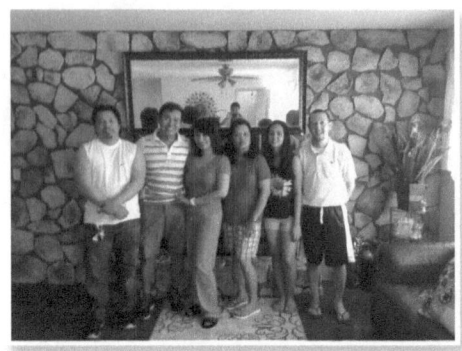

Joel's family with her classmate
Aisel & her husband

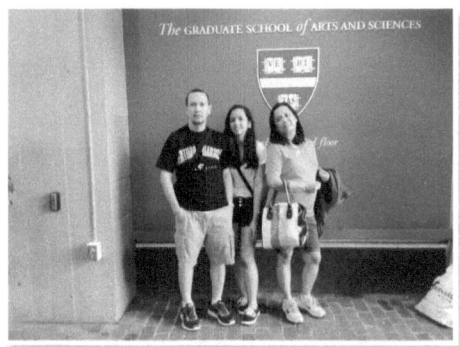

Joel & his family at Harvard School,
Cambridge, Massachusetts

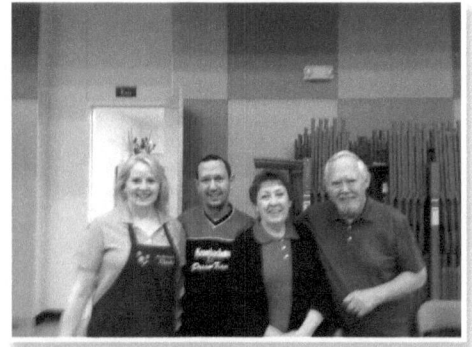

Joel & John with the
Women's Club sisters

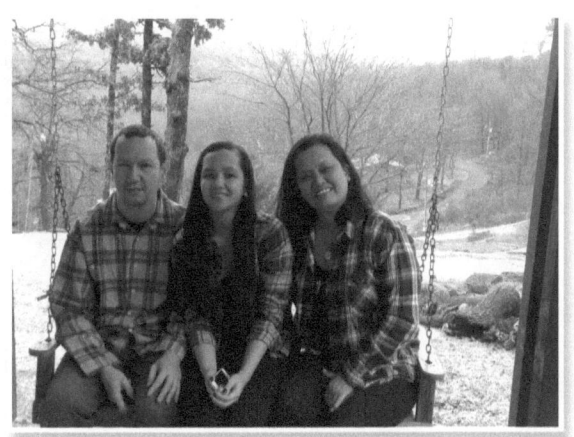

Joel & his family's Spring Break at
Lake Tenkiller, Oklahoma

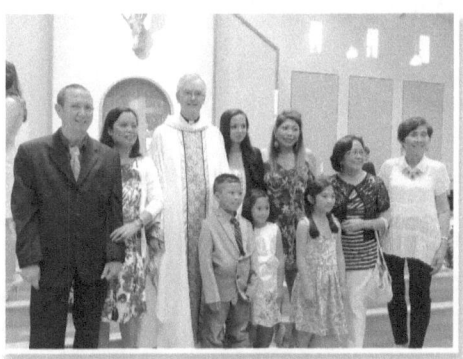

Joel & May's daughter
Krysha Confirmation with
Bishop Gregory Kelly

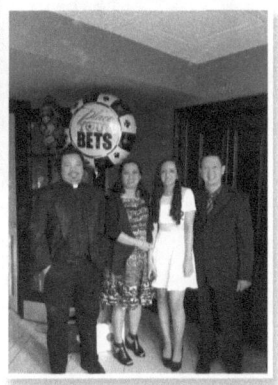

Joel's family with his
brother-in-law Fr. Cyrain
Cabuenas in New York

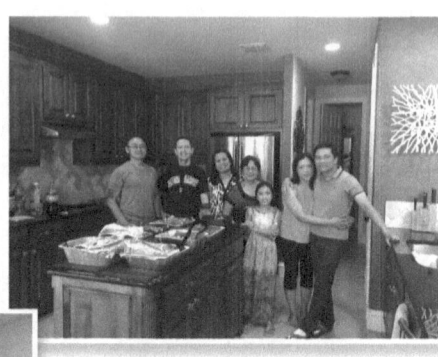

Joel & May with the Ramos
& Silverio family

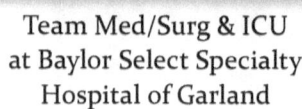

Team Med/Surg & ICU
at Baylor Select Specialty
Hospital of Garland

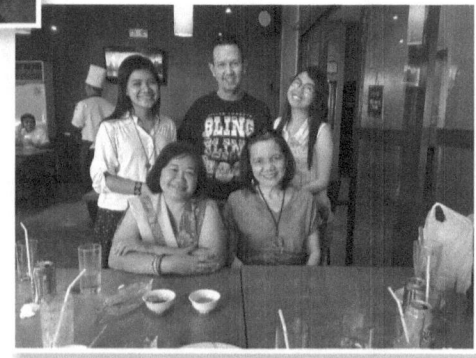

Joel with his fellow JVP Zamboanga
Local Community alumni

Plexus '90
25 Years and beyond

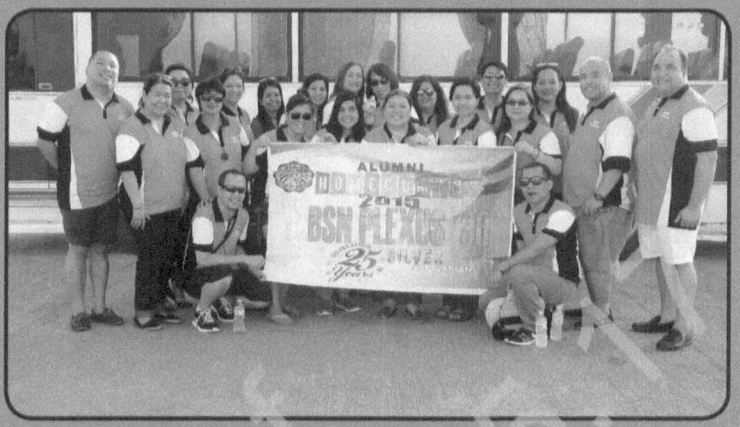

December 1-6, 2015
Zamboanga City, Phillipines

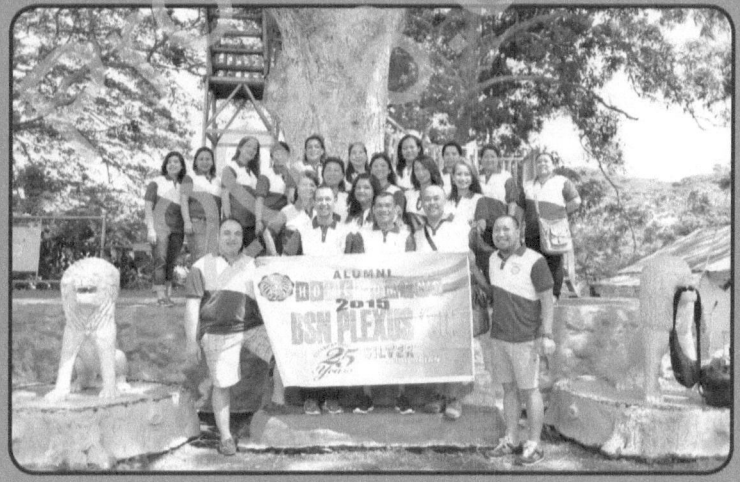

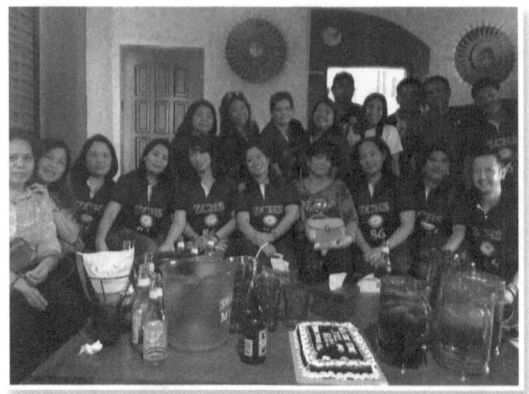

ZCHS Batch '86 reunion

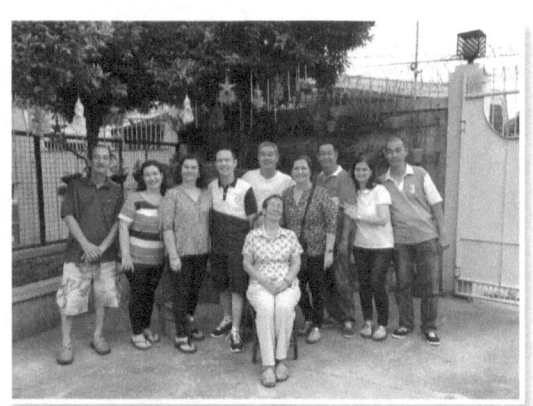

Joel with his mom & siblings

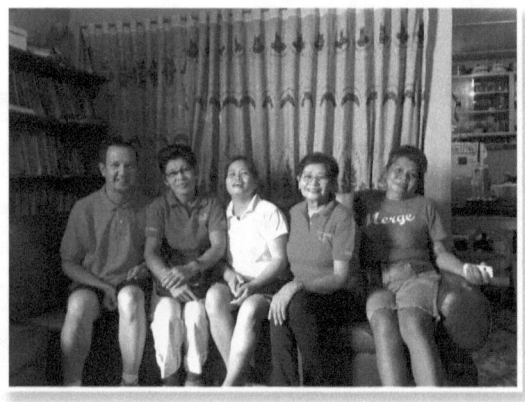

Joel with his aunts & cousins

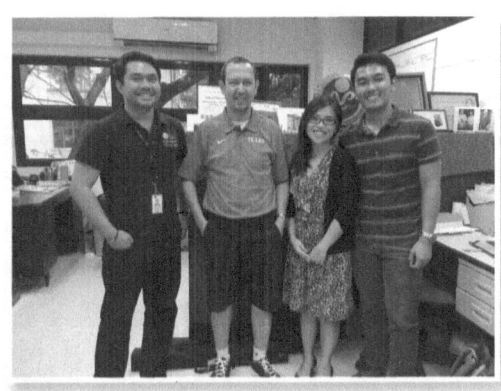

Joel with the JVPFI
central office staff

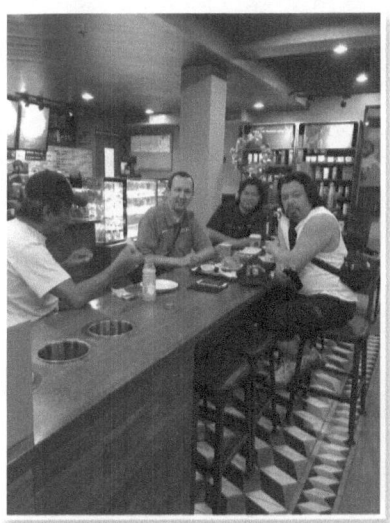

Joel with his two brothers-
in-law Fr. Cyrain & Fr.
Clyde, and uncle Cardo

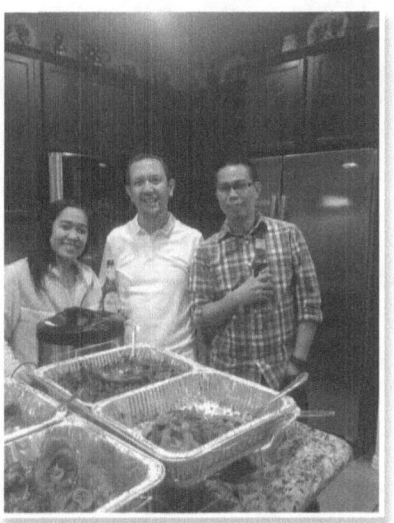

Joel with his fellow JVP
Manila housemates

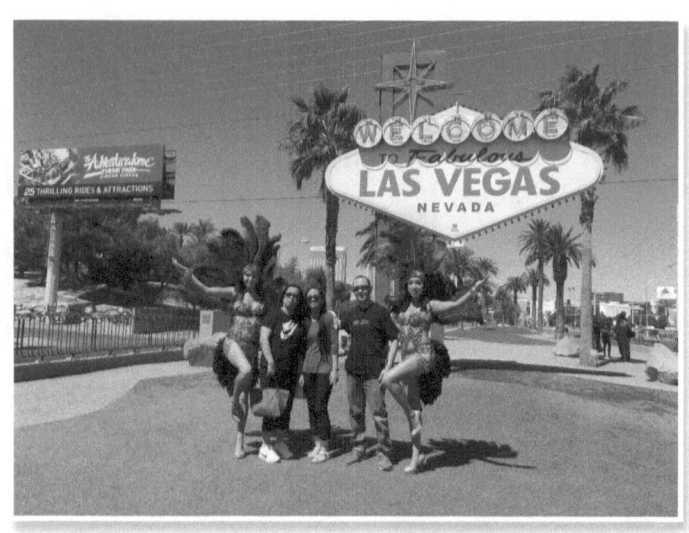

Joel & his family's Spring Break in Las Vegas

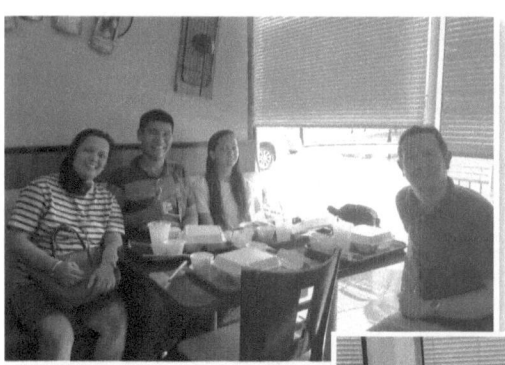

Joel & his family with his
nephew Lloyd Clemente

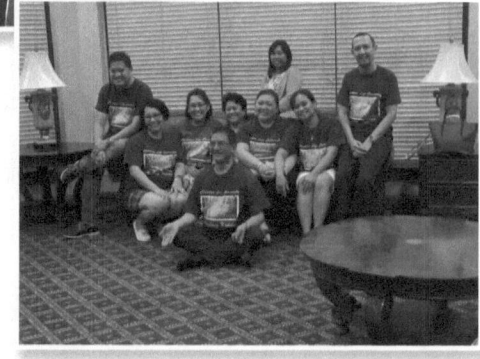

Angkong Kiddos reunion in Chicago,
Illinois with Fr. Denny Toledo, SJ

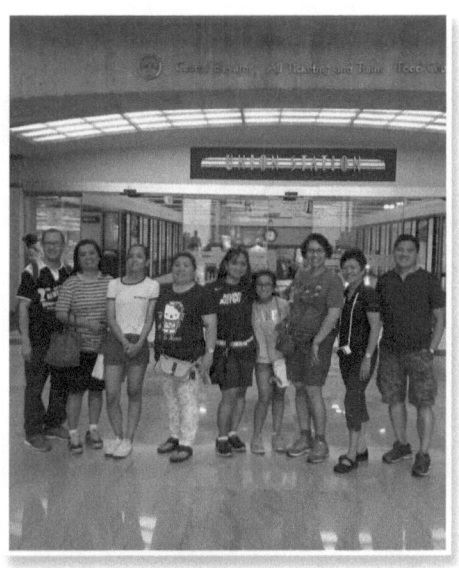

Angkong Kiddos reunion in Chicago,
Illinois with Fr. Denny Toledo, SJ

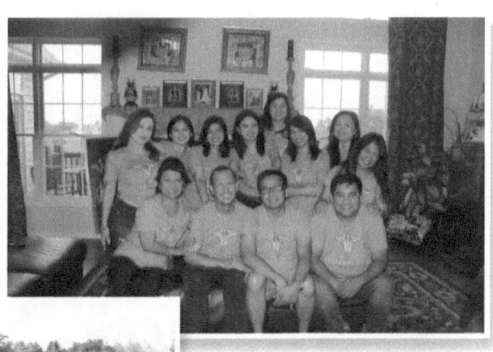

Plexus '90 26th
Anniversary
Class Reunion,
Chicago, Illinois

Plexus '90 26th Anniversary Class
Reunion, Chicago, Illinois

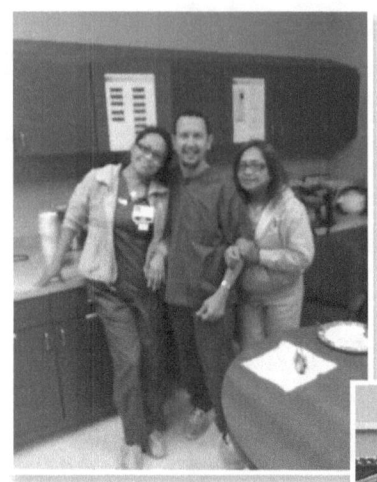

Team Med/Surg & ICU
at **Kindred Hospital
Dallas Central**

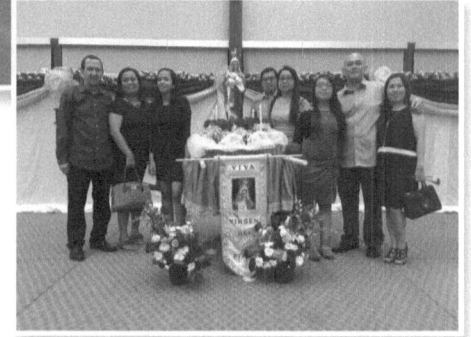

Zamboanga City Fiesta Pilar
celebration, Houston, Texas

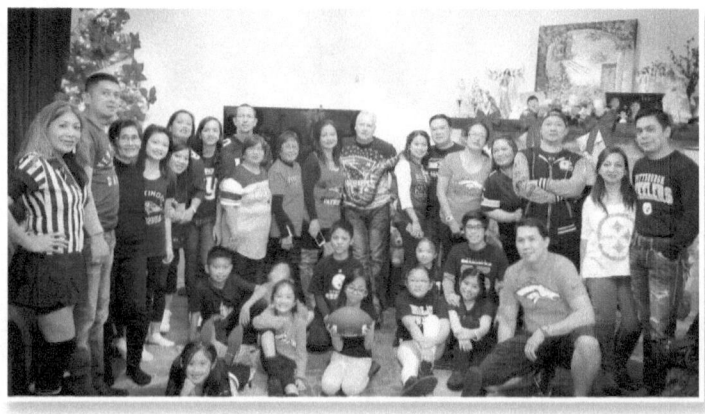

Joel with his fellow Pinoy @ Elite Westridge group

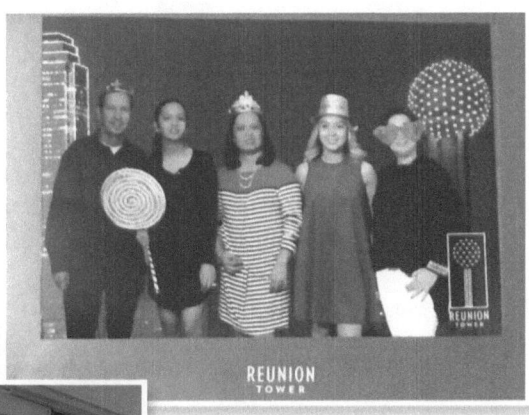

Joel's family with his
sister Jackie & his niece
at the Reunion Tower

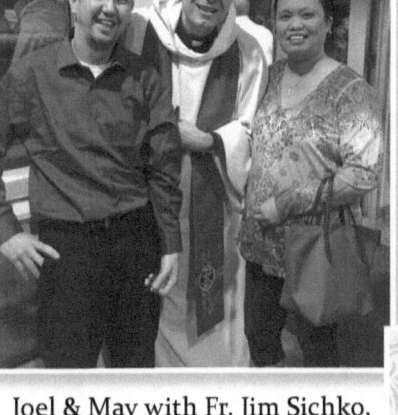

Joel & May with Fr. Jim Sichko,
author of "Among Friends
Stories from the Journey"

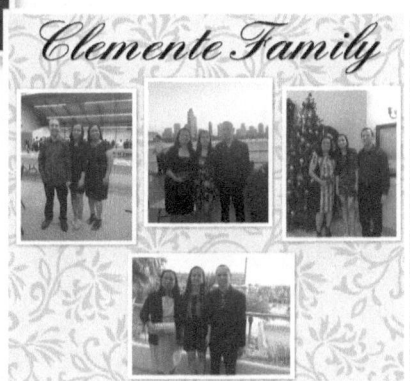

Clemente Family

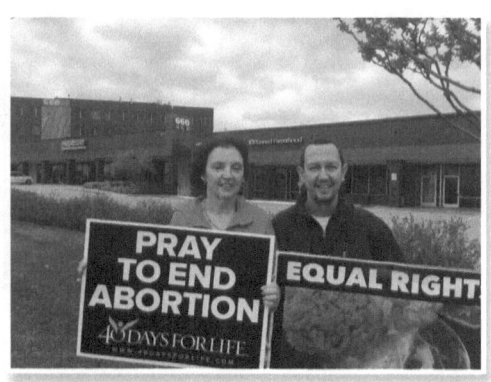

"40 Days For Life" prayer vigil
with Dan Kern & Rose Lorenz

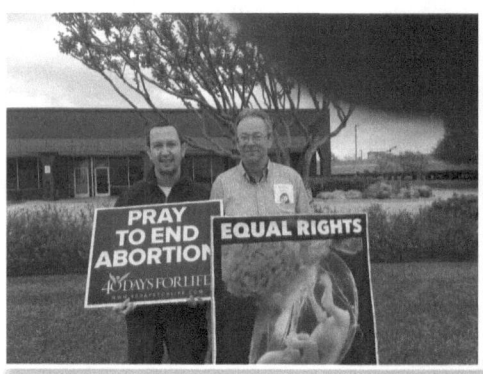

"40 Days For Life" prayer vigil
with Dan Kern & Rose Lorenz

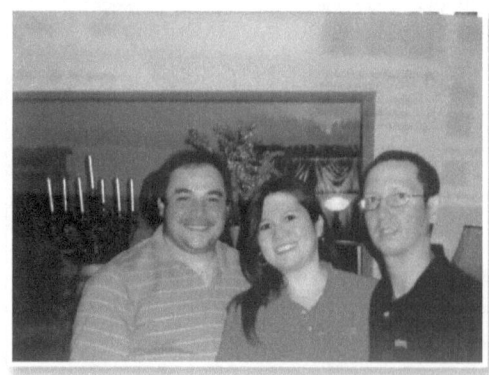

Joel with his classmates Lito Araneta
& Marilie Soliven-Nicandro

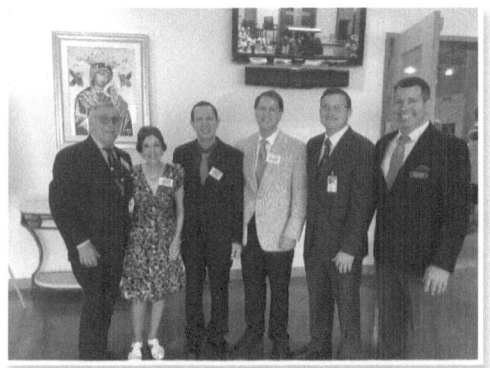

Joel with his fellow Hospitality
Ministry Team

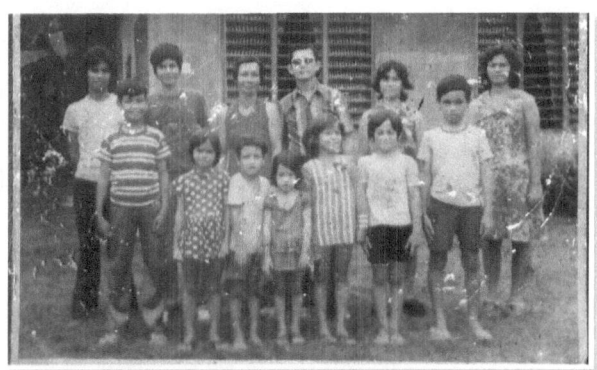

Joel with his parents & siblings circa 1970s

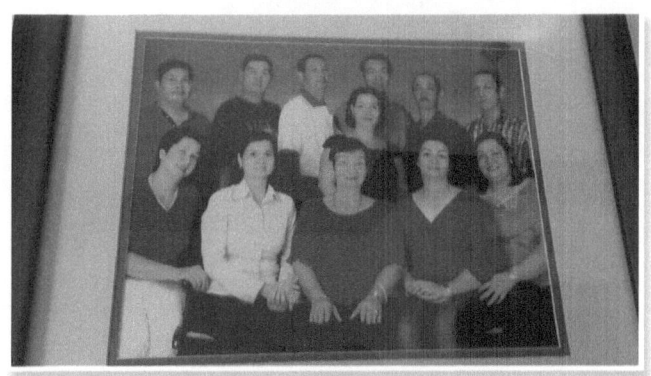

Joel with his mom & siblings
December 2005 family reunion

IN THE END

Now that you had read the story of my life and saw the photo gallery in this book, it is my fervent hope and prayers that in one way or other I had touched your life with what you read and ponder on the many pages of my work of art.

Thank you very much, God bless you all, and in the end I like to share with you Florante's song entitled *"Handog"* also known as "Offering."

> *Parang kailan lang ang mga pangarap ko'y kay hiram abutin*
> (Not so long ago, my dreams seemed too difficult to achieve)
> *Dahil sa inyo napunta ako sa aking nais marating*
> (Because of you, I was able to go where I wanted to)
> *Nais ko kayong pasalamatan kahit man lang sa isang awitin*
> (I want to thank you even with just one song)

Chorus

Tatanda at lilipas din ako

(I'll grow old and I'll be gone)

*Ngunit mayroong awiting iiwanan sa inyong
alaala*

(But there is a song I will leave for your memories)

Dahil minsan tayo'y nagkasama

(Because there was a time we had been together)

Based on Filipino singer and songwriter Florante De leon popularly known simply as *Florante* who wrote and sang the song in a Tagalog version during the 1970s per record of Wikipedia, the free encylopedia.

www.ingramcontent.com/pod-product-compliance
Lightning Source LLC
Chambersburg PA
CBHW030818180526
45163CB00003B/1335